What Is Schizophrenia?

William F. Flack, Jr.   Daniel R. Miller
Morton Wiener   Editors

What Is Schizophrenia?

Springer-Verlag
New York Berlin Heidelberg London Paris
Tokyo Hong Kong Barcelona Budapest

William F. Flack, Jr.
Department of Psychology
Frances L. Hiatt School of Psychology
Clark University
Worcester, MA 01610-1477
USA

Morton Wiener
Professor and Director of Clinical
    Training
Department of Psychology
Frances L. Hiatt School of Psychology
Clark University
Worcester, MA 01610-1477
USA

Daniel R. Miller
Department of Psychology
Frances L. Hiatt School of Psychology
Clark University
Worcester, MA 01610-1477
USA
and
Department of Psychology
Wesleyan University
Middletown, CT 06457
USA

Library of Congress Cataloging-in-Publication Data
What is schizophrenia? / William F. Flack, Jr., Daniel R. Miller,
    Morton Wiener, editors.
        p.   cm.
    Based on a conference sponsored by the Frances L. Hiatt School of
Psychology, at Clark University, Worcester, Mass., June 9–10, 1990.
    Includes bibliographical references and index.
    ISBN 0-387-97642-6 (alk. paper). — ISBN 3-540-97642-6 (alk.
paper)
    1. Schizophrenia — Congresses. I. Flack, William F.   II. Miller,
Daniel R.   III. Wiener, Morton.   IV. Frances L. Hiatt School of
Psychology.
    [DNLM: 1. Schizophrenia — congresses.   WM 203 W555 1990.]
RC514.W42   1991
616.89′82 — dc20
DNLM/DLC
for Library of Congress   91-4929

Printed on acid-free paper.

Camera-ready copy prepared by the editors.
Printed and bound by Edwards Brothers, Inc., Ann Arbor, MI.
Printed in the United States of America.

9 8 7 6 5 4 3 2 1

ISBN 0-387-97642-6 Springer-Verlag New York Berlin Heidelberg
ISBN 3-540-97642-6 Springer-Verlag Berlin Heidelberg New York

Acknowledgments and Dedication

The organization of even a relatively brief, two-day meeting such as ours takes much more effort than three organizers can muster even on their best days. Therefore, we want to thank the following individuals and groups for their crucial support and encouragement. First, we thank the Executive Committee of the Frances L. Hiatt School of Psychology for providing the funds which made both the conference and work on this book possible. We gratefully acknowledge the many helpful suggestions made by John Strauss, Courtenay Harding, and Jaak Rakfeldt, about our original proposal. For their support and technical assistance before, during, and after the conference, we thank Lorraine Cavallaro, Allison Jennings, and Michelle Regnier for their help that was generously given even in trying circumstances.

The staff of the Hiatt School also deserve recognition for their labors on our behalf. Natalie Acuna, Patricia Pulda, and Florence Resnick gave generously of their time and effort in assisting, coordinating, and teaching us about the many details attendant to organizing a conference. In particular, we are very appreciative of the painstaking work of Patrice Nash who, with the assistance of Kathy Sutton, managed the onerous task of dealing with seemingly endless revisions in the face of next-to-impossible deadlines.

We also express our heartfelt thanks to Manfred Bleuler, who provided a paper despite the taxing health problems which prevented him from attending the conference in person; and, in memoriam, to the late Joseph Zubin, whose level of energy and enthusiasm at the age of 90 were both astonishing and inspirational. Finally, we are sincerely appreciative of the authors cooperation, particularly their careful responses to our original questions and to our requests for revisions of their work.

This book is dedicated to Jacob Hiatt, benefactor of the Frances L. Hiatt School of Psychology at Clark University.

Contents

Contributors

Manfred Bleuler, Emeritus Prof. Dr. Med., University of Zurich, Switzerland.

Robert C. Carson, Professor of Psychology, Duke University, U.S.A.

Jeff Coulter, Professor of Sociology and Chair, Boston University, U.S.A.

Ruth Condray, Research Health Scientist, Biometric Research, Department of Veterans Affairs Medical Center; Instructor in Psychiatry, University of Pittsburg, School of Medicine, U.S.A.

Rue L. Cromwell, M. Erik Wright Distinguished Professor of Clinical Psychology, The University of Kansas, U.S.A.

Horacio Fabrega, Professor of Psychiatry and Anthropology, and Director of Medical Student Education, University of Pittsburgh School of Medicine, Western Psychiatric Institute and Clinic, U.S.A.

William F. Flack, Jr., Hiatt Fellow, Clark University, U.S.A.

Elliott Jaques, Visiting Research Professor of Management Science, George Washington University, U.S.A.

Bernard Kaplan, Professor of Psychology, Clark University, U.S.A.

Robert E. Kendell, Professor of Psychiatry and Dean, University of Edinburgh Medical School, Scotland.

Joseph Margolis, Professor of Philosophy, Temple University, U.S.A.

Paul R. McHugh, Henry Phipps Professor of Psychiatry, Director and Psychiatrist-in-Chief, The Johns Hopkins Medical Institutions, U.S.A.

Daniel R. Miller, Professor Emeritus of Psychology, Wesleyan University, and Research Professor of Psychology, Clark University, U.S.A.

Theodore R. Sarbin, Professor Emeritus of Psychology and Criminology, University of California at Santa Cruz, U.S.A.

Stuart R. Steinhauer, Director of Biometric Research, Department of
  Veterans Affairs Medical Center; Assistant Research Professor of
  Psychiatry, University of Pittsburgh, School of Medicine, U.S.A.

John S. Strauss, Professor of Psychiatry, Yale University School
  of Medicine, U.S.A.

Erik Strömgren, Professor of Psychiatry, Institute of Psychiatric
  Demography, Aarhus Psychiatric Hospital, Denmark.

Morton Wiener, Professor of Psychology and Director of Clinical
  Training, Clark University, U.S.A.

Joseph Zubin, Research Career Scientist, Biometric Research,
  Department of Veterans Affairs Medical Center; Distinguished Professor
  of Psychiatry, University of Pittsburgh, School of Medicine, U.S.A.

Introduction

William F. Flack, Jr., Daniel R. Miller, and Morton Wiener

What is schizophrenia?[1] This was the seemingly simple question posed to a diverse group of investigators asked to present their views at a conference sponsored by the Frances L. Hiatt School of Psychology at Clark University, Worcester, Massachusetts, in June, 1990. The plan was to have a small group of theoretically minded clinicians and investigators from different professions and orientations convene to discuss and debate conceptual and metatheoretical issues surrounding "schizophrenia." Instead of concentrating on the latest empirical findings, we were primarily interested in having a series of exchanges about the very different meanings and uses of this concept.[2]

In our review of the literature on schizophrenia, we uncovered what seemed to us to be multiple, non-overlapping uses of the term. For some investigators, it appears to be used to specify certain kinds of people; for others, it is employed to refer to certain kinds of behaviors. For still others, the term is grounded in biochemical events, or in socioculturally specific actions. A number of alternatives are explored in the contributors' papers in this volume.

Few investigators have pointed out the diversity of conceptions of schizophrenia; fewer still have observed that such differences constitute a problem for the field. For one, it is not at all clear that different investigators, utilizing different definitions, are working on the same problem, despite their use of the same term. Some usages of the term do not seem to be compatible with one another, even at the most basic level of what kinds of instances are to be identified. A related, and equally vexing problem is created by the different

---

[1]Given the diversity of usages and meanings in the different perspectives that follow, we will use the term schizophrenia in its most generic sense. We do not intend any specific meaning of the term, and would surround it with quotation marks in each instance save for the fact that it is unwieldy to do so.

[2]The heterogeneity of concepts should not be confused with the heterogeneity of clinical subtypes postulated in most standard nosologies (e.g., American Psychiatric Association, 1987). The former is rarely, if ever, considered; the latter is, by and large, taken for granted.

philosophies of science, paradigms, and disciplinary matrices in which the different usages of schizophrenia appear to be imbedded. The presumed agreement seems to have its roots in the use of a common term. In our postscript, we identify some apparent sources of differences in philosophical orientations.

In our original invitation to the contributors we asked them to discuss their conceptions of schizophrenia and the rationales underlying them. Drafts of the papers were circulated to all participants prior to the meetings so that authors needed only to present synopses of their arguments; the amount of time devoted to round-table discussions could be maximized. With the exception of two historical papers, by Manfred Bleuler and Joseph Zubin, each session consisted of three papers followed by a discussant's comments. This was followed by an open discussion. The sequence of papers in this volume follows that of the conference.

In contrast to some other conference reports, we decided not to include in this volume transcripts of the general discussions among the participants. No matter how interesting they may be, such verbatim transcriptions usually contain a very high ratio wheat to chaff. In light of the discussions we gave the participants the opportunity to revise their original drafts and comments for publication. Many of the ideas and controversies that were raised in round-table discussions appear in the following pages. As may be gleaned from these papers, many of the discussions, or more often, debates, were both intense and impassioned.

A brief word is in order about our choice of participants. To make a round-table format feasible, we opted for a small number of participants who could, we hoped, represent a fairly wide range of professional backrounds and orientations. We recognize, of course, that all potentially relevant frames of reference could not be represented at such a meeting. This particular group of participants was chosen primarily because of the significance of their earlier contributions, and their proclivities for addressing theoretical and metatheoretical issues in their writing. In addition, we were particularly interested in providing a forum in which individuals with very different perspectives would have opportunities to exchange opinions, explore commonalities, and explicate differences in points of view.

1
The Concept of Schizophrenia in Europe During the Past One Hundred Years

Manfred Bleuler

Schizophrenic Psychoses and Adolf Meyer's Common Sense Psychiatry

We are all confronted with a tragic fact: During their lives about 1% of the population become entirely different from the way they were before, and entirely different also from most of us. We are no longer able to understand much of what they say, think, and express emotionally. They change or neglect their usual activities. They become completely dependent on others. Frequently they no longer care if they live or die. Such alterations of the personality are enigmatic and mysterious because, as a rule, we are not able to discover the reasons for them. They cannot be explained either by damage to physical health, psychological stress, or a tragic fate. In spite of the loss of many important signs of being like the rest of us, these changed persons may, at times, demonstrate that they have quite normal human abilities that, as a rule, remain concealed.

Such tragic changes occur in some men and women in every society and culture we know of. We have good reason to believe that they also occurred in very ancient times. Some princes and kings also became victims of such a fate in previous centuries. Their conditions were described by their contemporaries in impressive detail. In the past, the disorder has been attributed to very different causes, such as obsession by the devil or by witches, or by the judgments of mysterious powers.

I have ventured to describe what we call schizophrenic psychoses in simple and popular words. It is good if we, as psychiatrists, are conscious of what the average man feels and if he is able to understand what we discuss in highly scientific language.

The consideration of what we now refer to as schizophrenic psychoses as a disease had already begun in some societies centuries ago. After the age of enlightenment, this idea became more and more common. At the beginning of the last century, great contributions in understanding schizophrenic psychoses from the medical point of view were made by French psychiatrists. During the present century, the schizophrenic psychoses were increasingly considered as diseases, and treated from a medical standpoint.

The present-day concept of schizophrenic psychoses goes back to the idea of "dementia praecox" of Emil Kraepelin (1899), theoretically conceived as a disease entity, and to the denomination "schizophrenic psychoses" of Eugen Bleuler (1911/1950). Bleuler's conception left open the question of whether or not schizophrenia was a disease entity. Rather, he wanted to express, with his term, the main characteristic of the disorder; that is, the dissociation, or splitting, of the patient's inner life.

More than one hundred years have passed since E. Kraepelin and E. Bleuler started to form their concepts of the psychoses during their early experiences in psychiatric hospitals. In venturing to summarize the origin of the concept of schizophrenic psychoses, and the development of our knowledge as regards them, for about one hundred years, *I am relying on my lifelong experience.* Eugen Bleuler, my father, told me much about his career-long experience of research on schizophrenics. Through him, I became acquainted with many prominent psychiatrists and their research on this problem. I myself was born in my father's psychiatric clinic, Burghölzli, spent all my youth there, and devoted a great part of my later life to my work in psychiatric clinics. A large part of my scientific research concerns the problems of schizophrenics. Although my experience with schizophrenics is, therefore, substantial, I must admit that it is one-sided. It is not based, for instance, on personal biochemical studies of brain function.

Eugen Bleuler's concept of schizophrenic psychoses was based first on his experience between 1886 and 1898 as a young man in the "Island Clinic of Rheinau." There he devoted all his time and interest to the care of his patients, and lived among them. He was their Doctor, and he treated them for a broad range of conditions, even performing operations half a day each week, both on his psychiatric patients and also, if urgent, on all the staff of the hospital and farmers in the neighborhood. However, his main endeavor was to be close to his patients; working with them, playing and walking with them, even organizing dancing parties with them. He became their friend, and they called him father. All this was because E. Bleuler was not yet married, had no family life in Rheinau, and had no social life outside the hospital, which was very isolated at that time. It was in Rheinau that he realized that schizophrenics could not be "demented" since they did not lose a lively and colorful inner life.

When Bleuler was appointed Professor of Psychiatry at the University of Zurich, and Head of the Zurich Clinic Burgholzli in 1898, he was very disappointed that he had to leave Rheinau. He changed his post because both his parents fell ill, and he could not visit them from Rheinau.

In Zurich, Bleuler elaborated his concept of schizophrenic psychoses in collaboration with the physicians of his Clinic. It has never been sufficiently realized how much the concept was influenced by his discussions with prominent psychiatrists of the time, such as Emil Kraepelin, Sigmund Freud, and Adolf Meyer. Bleuler knew each of them well, although the three had almost no contact with each other.[1]

It is one of Kraepelin's great merits that he refashioned psychiatry in the tradition of the natural sciences. One step in this direction was his introduction of the concept, "dementia praecox," following the nomenclature of Linne's classification of plants and animals, his "systema naturae." Eugen Bleuler had the greatest respect for Kraepelin's endeavors, but Bleuler felt the need to develop them further by studying schizophrenics more personally.

Bleuler initially became acquainted with Freud before he wrote on psychoanalysis, and followed the development of Freud's system with great interest. It was therefore natural that Bleuler would try to understand the ideas, delusions, hallucinations, and the whole inner life of schizophrenics in the way in which Freud developed his understanding of dreams and neuroses. Bleuler never carried out a prolonged psychoanalysis of a particular patient, but he analyzed many ideas and symptoms of schizophrenics. He discussed his findings personally with Freud, Jung, and all of his own pupils. He regretted, however, that they understood "only" the meaning of symptoms and ideas, but did not understand why their patients had become psychotic.

At that time, the problem was conceived as a morbid "process," hidden in the background of the schizophrenic's inner life, which was the real origin of the psychosis. Psychiatrists believed that they understood the symptoms, not the psychosis itself.

In his youth, Adolf Meyer had emigrated from Switzerland to the U.S.A. He became the best known American psychiatrist in the middle

---

[1]Freud and C.G. Jung met Adolf Meyer during a psychological conference held at Clark University in 1909.

decades of this century. I still remember very well one moment during his visits in Bleuler's clinic, although 65 years have passed since then. This episode clearly demonstrates Meyer's views on psychiatry, and his contribution to Bleuler's concept of schizophrenic psychoses. I accompanied Meyer and my father during a walk in the park of the clinic while the two of them discussed schizophrenic psychoses. Finally Bleuler remarked, "All we know is good to know, but now we should discover the 'primary process' which determines that psychological reactions result in a severe psychosis." At this point, Meyer got excited and said in a loud voice, "Spare me such hypothetical ideas of a process underlying the psychosis. Let us disregard speculations, and let us keep to what we see and observe." My father was profoundly impressed by this outburst. He concluded that we should continue to study everything we can observe with schizophrenic patients, but we should not waste time in looking for mysterious backgrounds of the psychosis. This was Meyer's (1948) common sense psychiatry. It helped Bleuler not to adhere too much to hypothetical ideas about a specific process underlying schizophrenic psychoses. It is interesting to note, in this regard, that such a process has not been found in the 65 years after Meyer's outburst.

The Result of Our Century's Research on Dementia Praecox and Schizophrenic Psychoses

Research on dementia praecox and schizophrenic psychoses has been significantly influenced by the terms themselves. The symptomatology of schizophrenic psychoses has been described in many textbooks, and this is not the place to repeat it. However, I shall mention some particular points. "Catatonia" and "catatonic symptoms," which were so well described by Kraepelin, have become increasingly rare, while paranoid and hebephrenic forms, and the so called "Schizophrenic simplex," are more frequent. It is probable that modern care for patients has created such a change. When one watched, however, as I have, the shift in interest of many psychiatrists within the past decades, another explanation for such a change seems possible. For a long time, catatonic symptoms, such as catalepsy, stupor, stereotypy of movements and speech, mannerisms, and so on, were the most fascinating signs of schizophrenic psychoses. There were professors of psychiatry who were eager to demonstrate the impressive catatonic signs to their students, and less interested in speaking with the patients or demonstrating their manners of thinking and feeling. It is good that this has changed, and it raises the interesting question of the degree to which the symptoms observed in schizophrenics have been dependent on the interests of their psychiatrists. Did it change the patient's symptomatology, for instance, if the psychiatrist was fascinated by demonstrating catatonic symptoms, and not interested in speaking empathically with the patient?

Within the last decades, a better general view has slowly been gained of schizophrenics' various symptoms. On one hand, no particular mental function is lost for good during schizophrenic psychoses. On the other hand, schizophrenic mental life is characterized by an important loss of sufficient coherence in thinking, feeling, and acting. Thoughts, feelings, and actions frequently arise independently of other thoughts and feelings. In particular, there is often a lack of adapting parts of the inner life to experience, to critical evaluations, and to logical thinking. Again, logical thinking is not lost forever and in every respect, but, nonetheless, in many important ways. This general view justifies the designation "schizophrenic psychosis;" that is, psychosis characterized at times by a split inner life, by a lack of psychological harmony.

Course and Outcome

In regard to the course and outcome of schizophrenic psychoses, long-standing research, in which I have participated for over 60 years, has confirmed what was doubted for a long time. *There is no specific course* for the disorder (Bleuler, 1978; Ciompi, 1984). Instead, the outcomes of schizophrenic psychoses are extremely diverse, varying among prolonged recovery, intermittent course, and prolonged psychosis of severe or mild degrees. For a long time, many psychiatrists believed that a precise definition of the diagnosis indicated a specific prognosis.[2] Experience has shown that no matter how we formulate the diagnosis; it never insures predictable course and outcome.

An impressive experience for all of us is discovering in every schizophrenic patient the chance to know well a lively, colorful inner life. Rather new is the discovery that even manifold artistic abilities persist or, in fact, become evident in schizophrenics.

The course of schizophrenic psychoses never goes in the direction of increasing impoverishment of inner life, never towards a "dementia"

---

[2]Within recent times, such an assumption has been called "Neo-Kraepelinian." This is wrong. Kraepelin never tried to disregard facts, even those which were contradictory to his early hypothesis that dementia praecox was a disease entity with specific course and outcome. He himself described long-standing recoveries of patients he considered suffering from dementia praecox.

of the type found in cases of diffuse brain damage. The inner life may be hidden by lack of expression, in mutism, for example, but it is not lost.[3]

The collection of statistical data on the course and outcome of schizophrenic psychoses is fairly new. The lack of knowledge became particularly troublesome at the time when treatment with repeated hypoglycaemic episodes, caused by injection of insulin, were common.[4] In attempting to evaluate the results of insulin treatment, psychiatry was confronted with the embarrassing "discovery" that the outcome of schizophrenic psychoses without insulin treatment was problematic. At this time, some unrealistic suppositions were formulated that today seem almost absurd. It was maintained, for instance, that there was "never any recovery of a schizophrenic psychosis without insulin," but that "with insulin, every schizophrenic patient recovers."

The more precise knowledge we have today started with long-term studies in Switzerland, Germany, and the U.S.A. (Bleuler, 1978; Ciompi, 1984; Huber et al., 1980; Muller & Ciompi, 1976). These results have been confirmed recently by large-scale studies in the U.S.A., such as the "Vermont Study" (Harding et al., 1987), as well as in other countries. Their results are easily summarized. Between 20 and 25% of schizophrenics recover for many years, probably for the rest of their lives. About one half of the remaining patients show a very variable course, such as acute psychotic episodes interspersed with improved or even good periods. The other half remain in a fairly mild psychotic condition for the rest of their lives. They can be cared for by their families, or in open homes or open hospitals.

It has not been shown that these outcome statistics have been changed with new therapies such as the use of neuroleptics. Some of these new therapies do improve the actual condition of many patients. However, they hardly improve the number of long-lasting recoveries, nor diminish the number of chronic psychoses.

Origin of Schizophrenic Psychoses

As for the origin of schizophrenic psychoses, we must openly confess

---

[3]Self-evident exceptions are those cases where a schizophrenic psychosis is complicated by a severe cerebral disease; for instance, Alzheimer's disease, in which case "dementia" is a complicating factor.

[4]This treatment had been introduced by Sakel in 1933, and was often applied in the years prior to the introduction of neuroleptics in the 1950s.

that even the considerable research of the last 100 years has not produced the discovery of a specific cause. It seems probable that such a cause does not exist. This fact has disappointed many psychiatrists. Notwithstanding the lack of positive results, such research has been organized along the following three lines.

1. Study of the Nature and Origin of a Disposition to Schizophrenic Psychoses

Manifold and numerous peculiarities of somatic, physiological, and psychological natures have been identified as causes of vulnerability to schizophrenic psychoses. Some are inherited, others acquired, and in many of them there is an interaction of heredity and experience. The discoveries consist in demonstrating that the peculiarities in question were significantly more common in schizophrenics before the onset of the psychosis than in the general population. We should remain conscious of one fact which it would be pleasant to forget; namely, that none of the peculiarities considered today as dispositions are present in all schizophrenics either before or after the outbreak of the psychosis. They can also be found in some normal people, or in many patients other than schizophrenics. In short, this means that we have not discovered any *specific* dispositions for schizophrenic psychoses.

It is bewildering to consider the great number of such dispositions that have been posited and of what extremely diverse nature they are. In modern times, the number of these discoveries is increasing to an astonishing degree. Some concern the general body build, or some other peculiarities. These were already known at the beginning of the century as so called "signs of degeneration."[5] The dysplastic and asthenic body constitutions were described well by Kretschmer (1925). The description of pathologies of the cerebral ventricles by Huber and others (Gross, Huber, & Schuttler, 1982) led to many discoveries of the cerebral structures of schizophrenics. After establishing that neuroleptics influencing the psychosis also influenced the cerebral hormonal metabolism, researchers began to look for cerebro-hormonal dispositions for schizophrenia.

Characterological dispositions for schizophrenia were also described very early on. The first important one was Kretschmer's (1956) description of the "schizoid personality." By this he meant people with

---

[5]At one time, schizophrenic psychoses themselves were characterized as "degenerative."

a rich inner life, but with difficulties in making emotional contact with others, and with abundant intrapsychic problems.

In recent times, there have been identified some particular psychological predispositions for schizophrenia. Within the past few decades, much research was carried out on the relationships of adult schizophrenics during their childhoods with their mothers, fathers, and the whole family. It is certain now that troublesome attitudes expressed by the parents to the future patient play an important role.

Until a few decades ago, a distinction was made between psychological and somatic dispositions for schizophrenic psychoses. There was even a tendency to consider somatic predispositions as a sign of somatic backgrounds of schizophrenic psychoses, and characterological and intrapsychic dispositions as a sign of psychological background. Such sharp distinctions have vanished today, as most of the somatic dispositions are now known to influence potentially the psychic development and life. Astonishing in this regard is the discovery of "neuronal plasticity," the possibility that life experience might change the cerebral structure, in particular the communication between neurons. It is tempting to state that somatic peculiarities frequently influence the psychic life and can frequently represent dispositions for a schizophrenic psychosis. We must also take into account that our inner life influences the cerebral structures.

I have pointed out many and various signs of disposition to schizophrenic psychoses. To enumerate all of them does not lie within the scope of this paper. I have tried, however, to mention some of them to demonstrate their tremendous variability, which is often neglected. Such a discussion yields impressive results. In spite of their tremendous variability, all of the dispositions for schizophrenic psychoses can have one essential effect in common. They render the formation and the preservation of a harmonious personality difficult. This has been carefully described with respect to the so called "double-bind," in which contradictory emotional attitudes to parents are created by contradictory experiences with them. It is self-evident that disharmonic body structures have an influence in the same way, that, for instance, an infantile form of the body of an intellectually and emotionally mature man or woman make for great difficulty in being a well-harmonized man or woman. Many cerebral structural or physiological peculiarities have been discovered which can act in the same manner.[6]

In short, the schizophrenic is characterized by his split,

---

[6]For instance, an imbalance between structures and functions of the left and right hemispheres of the brain.

unharmonious inner life. What predisposes him to become schizophrenic are just those peculiarities which promote disharmony of the personality. This becomes evident during prolonged psychotherapy of difficult persons who later become schizophrenic. When we are able to become acquainted with the past of our schizophrenic patients, we are frequently impressed to discover that they have really struggled before the beginning of the psychosis with their contradictory inner existence.

2. Study of the Circumstances to Which the Beginning of the Psychosis is Due

On what occasion does a vulnerable person become schizophrenic? The answer suggests itself if we know the patient's difficulties before he became psychotic. The psychosis breaks out when the fight for overcoming the inner difficulties becomes too difficult or impossible. If we are in close touch with our patients during the course of psychotherapy, the truth of such an answer is evident.

There are, however, also many other experiences which illustrate the role of vulnerability. A not infrequent example is that of a woman who falls sick from a schizophrenic psychosis soon after the birth of her first child. The study of her past shows that her mother had never expressed warm maternal feelings towards her offspring, and that she was, therefore, afraid of becoming a mother herself. She had feared that she would not be a real mother of her own child, even though she wanted with all her heart to be one. Confronted with her newborn child and the duties of a mother, she could no longer endure this inner conflict. She gave up her fight to overcome the inner contradiction, and became schizophrenic.

The tragic confrontation with inner contradictions, however, is not the only trigger for a schizophrenic psychosis. Quite a different kind is the change in mood caused by other than psychological reasons. Manic-depressive psychoses and, more frequently, mild mood swings, in the sense of elation or depression, are frequent at the outbreak of a schizophrenic psychosis or of a schizo-affective psychosis. For this reason, we can also understand another statistical finding; that among the parents of schizophrenics there are more affective psychoses than in the general population. The reason for this is that mood swings in people vulnerable to schizophrenia cause the outbreak of schizophrenic psychoses, while schizophrenic episodes never give rise to manic-depressive psychoses.

3. Study of Influences on the Course and Outcome of the Psychoses

What affects the course and outcome of schizophrenic psychoses? Our medical therapy plays a great role, which I shall discuss later. Apart from medical therapy, it is evident that social conditions greatly influence the fate of schizophrenics. There are societies which do not care sufficiently for agitated or quite passive schizophrenic patients, and neglect them to such a degree that many of them die. At various times, and in some societies, many schizophrenics have been treated with extreme cruelty, and even killed. However, there are also some social traditions which are beneficial for some or many schizophrenics. In some societies, a few severely sick schizophrenics are highly honored hermits. For many people, it is natural to feed them and to do everything possible for them. Even centuries ago, many psychotics were cared for in monasteries, and the course of their psychoses were mild under such care.

Our Present Concept of Therapy of Schizophrenic Patients

I will now give a short survey of our present concept of therapy of schizophrenic patients. It is not, of course, the place here to discuss therapeutic details such as, for instance, newly introduced neuroleptics. I will, however, point out the most important general conclusions based on a century of our therapy.

A specific therapy for schizophrenia has not been discovered. Every therapy that helps schizophrenics also helps many other sick patients, and there is no therapy for schizophrenics that is solely responsible for a long-standing recovery. We can summarize this experience in a formula that is wise and has come into common use. Namely, it is not the task of the physician to treat a sickness called "schizophrenia," rather it is his task to treat a schizophrenic patient. One of the consequences of this way of thinking is that the physician must know his schizophrenic patient personally. He has to stay near him. This important truth is often neglected, for instance, when the ability of a psychiatrist to be personally near the patient is not taught by psychiatric academicians or encouraged by directors of psychiatric hospitals.

The temptation to believe in the specificity of one or another treatment of schizophrenics has been great during our century, a temptation I have already referred to concerning insulin treatment. Another example occurred two decades later, when the action of neuroleptics on the cerebral dopamine metabolism became suggestive of a specific action, another idea that has been disproved.

The therapy that has proved to be useful consists essentially in caring for the patient in an appropriate way; in a hospital, therapeutic community, or at home. The distinction between caring for the patient and treating the patient is inappropriate in the light of modern experience. Caring in an appropriate way for the patient has been found to be the best therapy.

Good and steady relationships with other men or women, which are friendly and cordial, but not emotionally overloaded, are important in organizing care for the patient. In some cases, the physician called in for help is the first person with whom such a relationship can be achieved. In many other cases, family therapy can aid in attaining good relationships with family members. There are many other relationships of therapeutic significance, such as the relationships with companions at work, or those fighting for the same idealistic aims as the patient. In some cases, relationships within a religious circle prove to be helpful.

Just as important is the case for steady work for schizophrenic patients. In acute phases of the disease, this is hardly possible, but even the most primitive occupations are helpful when others are not possible. Here I would like to mention an experience in old psychiatric hospitals. In those days, male patients participated in groups in farming around the hospital, and many female patients took part with nurses in cooking and caring for the household of the hospital. In this way, therapeutic groups were formed that were often of value. They can hardly be formed in the old ways in our time, but new possibilities exist in constructing groups around mutual occupations and for the purpose of forming healthy relationships.

Long-standing personal psychotherapy, in the strict sense of the word, is, in many cases, of impressive significance. In the course of such treatment, the therapist gains insight into the background of his patient's inner life, understands it in the same way that we understand other people and our own inner life, and can feel with them as we feel with healthy people. Such experiences have a significant impact on the therapist, and are of great help for many patients.[7] The patient can be helped, encouraged, and touched by the therapist's intellectual understanding of his morbid life, and by his ability to feel with him. For evident reasons, it is not possible to organize very long psychotherapies with this aim for all of our patients, but even shorter and less intensive treatments may have a similar effect.

---

[7]Such experiences have been described, for instance, by Benedetti (1985).

Pharmacotherapy for schizophrenics, mainly with "neuroleptics," is of great help to many patients if the physician realizes the dangers of these drugs, restricts their application and the dosage as far as possible, and watches the patient closely for unwelcome or dangerous side-effects. Neuroleptic medications improve the patient's condition under many circumstances; in particular, when he shows agitation or when he is feeling agitated, even when not demonstrating it outwardly. In many other cases, neuroleptics protect a patient from repeated recurrences after recoveries.

More common at the beginning of this century than nowadays, "fatal catatonia" was the term used for death associated with a severe schizophrenic agitation. It was characterized not only by great agitation, but also by increasing exhaustion, excitation, and fever without demonstrable causes. It has always been difficult to determine whether the deaths of catatonics after their great agitation were due to the therapies, such as hypnotics, insulin comas, and electroshocks, that had been applied. With today's therapies, these deaths have become much rarer. However, one question which has not been studied sufficiently is the extent to which the severe neuroleptic syndrome is related to deaths considered to be caused by catatonia.

What can we think of the effects of our therapies for schizophrenics? Our experience is very *encouraging*. We can improve most schizophrenic conditions with neuroleptics, as well as diminish or even prevent, relapses in cases of schizophrenia with intermittent course. With good care of our patients, including psychotherapy and social therapies, we can diminish the neuroleptic treatments, or, in many cases, care for the patient without them. Under the influence of appropriate psychotherapy and care in open hospitals and open, well-organized homes for schizophrenics, most of them can live a fair life and, in the main, are content with this life. This means much if we consider the terrible fate of many schizophrenics in prisons or in some prison-like overfilled institutions. Before the introduction of current care and therapies, many, although not all, schizophrenics were a terrible burden for their families, and especially for their children. Such misery has been lessened by present-day care.

Given my positive remarks about modern care for schizophrenics, it is perhaps embarrassing to recall that I have also stated that modern therapy does not affect the numbers of long-standing complete recoveries or of chronic severe psychoses. Indeed, our available statistics indicate that the percentage of stable, full recoveries are between 20 and 25%, and that this percentage did not change after the introduction of new medical therapies, including neuroleptics. Despite such a statement, the results of our present care for schizophrenics are encouraging. The great majority of schizophrenics suffer far less than in former times, and most of them are able to recover the feeling that they are, again, the natural personality that they once were. They are able to feel closer to their families, friends, and comrades, and they also feel nearer to us, their physicians, than in previous times.

One observation that lends support to these hopeful statements is that many schizophrenics who in former days could only be cared for in closed wards of overfilled asylums today live quietly and fairly well in open wards or in open institutions, in family-like surroundings. In addition, many other schizophrenics who formerly would have had repeated psychotic episodes after initial improvements, are today, under good medical and social care, practically recovered.[8]

Other Findings of Importance

For the lack of space, I have had to omit several contributions to this summary of a century's psychiatric research with schizophrenic patients. These are outlined briefly below.

One is that since the beginning of our century, manifold and important studies have been conducted concerning the health of the relatives of schizophrenic patients, research in which I have participated for decades. While the average number of schizophrenics among relatives is well known, the general conclusions have not been considered sufficiently until quite recently. The psychiatric morbidity of relatives of schizophrenics is essentially the same in all societies and at all times during which it has been investigated. I have studied the rates of morbidity, in what was at that time the rather isolated mountain valleys of Tamina, in the Swiss cities of Basle and Zurich, and among relatives of patients in a private hospital in White Plains, New York. I have also followed many family pedigrees back until the beginning of the last century. One of the findings from this work is that the psychiatric morbidity of relatives of schizophrenics has remained about the same in different cultures and at different times. This might be a hint that the essential backgrounds of schizophrenic psychoses lie more in human nature than in particular troubles.

A second contribution to recent knowledge is that no Mendelian kind of heredity has been discovered for schizophrenia. For instance, the fact that the rate of occurrence of schizophrenic psychoses in children and siblings of schizophrenics is about the same constitutes

---

[8]In spite of their happier lives, these individuals are not counted statistically as "totally recovered" because their need for medical prophylactic treatment proves that their recovery is not total.

an argument against Mendelian heredity. An additional contribution from research on heredity has come from the study of twins of whom only one became schizophrenic. The results of this work indicate that hereditary and environmental influences together play an important part in the genesis of schizophrenia.

A third contribution whose implications have not yet been fully explored comes from a new field of research in physics called "synergetics." Investigators working with these ideas, also referred to as *Chaos theory*, study conditions characterized by the loss of coherence between the different components of a physical system. The physical chaos need not last forever. Order, or coherence, may suddenly be re-established. Peter Waser is credited with having suggested that the chaos theory can be compared with the theory that the splitting, the incoherence of different parts of our inner lives may be the background of schizophrenic psychoses.

Summary

Now at the end of this paper, I shall venture to summarize briefly the experience and research of the last one hundred years, that is, since Emil Kraepelin and Eugen Bleuler started to study the tragic phenomenon that they called "dementia praecox" and "schizophrenic psychoses."

At the end of the present century, the main background of, or disposition toward, schizophrenic psychoses, can be considered in a different light. Our vulnerability to schizophrenic psychoses is rooted in our rich, multifarious, colorful, grand inner life. Because of its richness and abundance, it also contains manifold contradictions, among different conclusions, our daily life experiences, and our present and past experiences. It is a continual and great task for all of us to overcome these contradictions, to come to conclusions in spite of arguments for and against them, to have a convincing emotional attitude. In short, to harmonize our inner life.

At the beginning of this paper, I mentioned some of the influences which make inner harmonization especially difficult. They are of the most varying kinds, and many have much to with heredity, whereas others are mostly due to psychological or social peculiarities.

The difficulties in overcoming our inner contradictions, in being a harmonized personality, become, in certain men and women, so painful, so insurmountable, that they abandon the fight for harmonization in various and important spheres of their inner lives. From this moment on, their thoughts, emotions, attitudes, and actions are split, dissociated, in a word, *schizophrenic*.

What are the possibilities for helping schizophrenic patients? They consist mainly of the same influences that help all of us from early childhood on to be "one of us," to be integrated into our societies and our worlds, and to be active in accordance with our interests, emotional attitudes, and personalities. The physician can help his patient to organize his life according to his needs, and by choosing the therapy suitable for the individual patient. To be able to do all of this, he needs to know his patient personally, and to stay near him.

References

Benedetti, G. (1985).   Meine entwicklung in der schizophrenietherapie. *Schweitzer Archiv für Neurologie, Neurochirurgie, und Psychiatrie, 136*(1), 23-28.

Bleuler, E. (1911/1950). *Dementia praecox or the group of schizophrenias.* NY: International Universities Press.

Bleuler, M. (1978). *The schizophrenic disorders: Long-term patient and family studies.* New Haven, CT: Yale University Press.

Ciompi, L. (1984). Is there really a schizophrenia? The long term course of psychotic phenomena. *British Journal of Psychiatry, 145,* 636-640.

Gross, G., Huber, G., & Schuttler, R. (1982). Computerized tomography studies on schizophrenic diseases. *Archiv für Psychiatrie und Nervenkrankheiten, 231*(6), 519-526.

Harding, C.M., Brooks, G.W., Ashikaga, T., Strauss, J.S., & Breier, A. (1987). The Vermont longitudinal study of persons with severe mental illness, I.: Methodology, study sample, and overall status 32 years later. *American Journal of Psychiatry, 144,* 718-726.

Huber, G., Gross, G., Schuttler, R., & Linz, M. (1980). Longitudinal studies of schizophrenic patients. *Schizophrenia Bulletin, 6*(4), 592-605.

Kraepelin, E. (1899). *Psychiatrie: Ein lehrbuch for studiende und aertze, 6te.* Leipzig: J.A. Barth.

Kretschmer, E. (1925). *Physique and character: An investigation of the nature of constitution and of the theory of temperament* (translated from the second, revised and enlarged edition by W.J.H. Sprott). NY: Harcourt, Brace & Company.

Kretschmer, E. (1956). *Medizinische psychologie.* Stuttgart: G. Thieme.

Meyer, A. (1948). *The common sense psychiatry.* NY: McGraw-Hill.

Muller, C. & Ciompi, L. (1976). The relationship between anamnestic factors and the course of schizophrenia. *Comprehensive Psychiatry, 17*(3), 387-393.

2

Schizophrenia from an American Perspective

Joseph Zubin[1], Stuart R. Steinhauer, and
Ruth Condray

The theme of this volume is the search for a definition of schizophrenia which would encompass its essence, i.e., arrive at the core nature of this disorder. This raises a philosophical and semantic issue, namely, what is the purpose of defining such concepts as schizophrenia, and what are the tests of its value. The possible options open to us are answers to the following questions: (1) does such a definition exist; (2) is it a true definition; (3) is it a useful definition? As to whether schizophrenia exists: what can be said with conviction? Conventional wisdom can help us here, and its answer would probably be yes, given the fact that schizophrenia runs in families and that it has a certain reliability regarding age of onset. Outcome would lead one to accept its existence in a pragmatic way. As Seymour Kety once said, "If it is a myth, it is a myth with a strong genetic component." Whether we can define it in such a way that it will be true is debatable, but the usefulness of a concept is possibly as important as its truth value. Even if its truth has not been established, it is still acceptable if its usefulness can be demonstrated for the purposes of classification, treatment, and communication. The question of whether or not we can arrive at its essence raises the problem identified by Aristotle, who claimed that every category has an essence. However, schizophrenia may have more than one essence, for, as Wittgenstein has asserted, the fact that a thing has only one name does not mean that it is only one thing. That a tree is a thing is

---

[1]Joseph Zubin died quietly on December 18, 1990 at the age of 90. His colleagues wish to acknowledge his teaching and mentoring to students of psychopathology from a variety of professional disciplines, and his enthusiastic pursuit of knowledge. The major contributions of this paper were made by Dr. Zubin.

Preparation of this paper was supported by the Medical Research Service of the Department of Veterans Affairs and by NIMH Grants MH43615 and MH45331.

generally accepted, but its significance varies with the aspect of the tree that is of interest, and this can vary with whether it is being considered by a house owner, an environmentalist, a forester, a lumberman, a landscaper, or a tree surgeon (who considers whether it is vulnerable to disease). The degree of rigor required for our definition of schizophrenia is debatable. Pertinent to our problem is Huxley's discussion about defining a species:

> There is no single criterion of species. Morphological difference; failure to interbreed; infertility of offspring; ecological geographical, or genetical distinctness—all those must be taken into account, but none of them singly is decisive. Failure to interbreed or to produce fertile offspring is the nearest approach to a positive criterion. It is, however, meaningless in apogamous forms, and as a negative criterion it is not applicable, many obviously distinct species, especially of plants, yielding fertile offspring, often with free Mendelian recombination in crossing. A combination of criteria is needed, together with some sort of flair (Huxley, 1940, p. 11).

When we realize that there is no singular definition of species in biology, and yet biology flourishes, we may lower our demand for absolute conceptual rigor for a definition of schizophrenia, lest too much rigor bring on rigor mortis. Since we have not yet identified the etiology of schizophrenia, we must be satisfied with an ad hoc operational definition "subject to change" without notice, as some travel schedules warn. Despite the above considerations, we have been asked to present an American view of schizophrenia as a complement to the European views presented in this volume by Professor Manfred Bleuler.

We have the advantage of having read beforehand Manfred Bleuler's intimate description of the development of his concept of schizophrenia, and our presentation shows its influence. He described how his father, Eugen, transmitted his views to him directly, and also how he learned these views indirectly through observing his father's interactions with his friends Emil Kraepelin, Adolf Meyer and Sigmund Freud. He distilled this intellectual inheritance through his own experience as a life-long friend of his patients and their families, and as a "caretaker" rather than as a "therapist." That is why his view is so unique and precious.

You will now be able to compare how Manfred Bleuler developed his concept and how we, 3,000 miles away, one of us a Lithuanian immigrant to the United States, developed ours. To our great surprise we arrived at a common understanding, though both concepts represent what as recently as a generation ago was perceived to be a maverick view when compared to the views of the establishment in both our cultures. The differences that do exist between Manfred Bleuler and us are largely due to the differences in our approaches. Bleuler uses the clinical method, whereas we use the biometric method, namely, the application of measurement to the clinically intuitive, subjective, and sometimes amorphous concepts that are still the basic conceptual underpinnings of the disorder. But what is the difference between the biometric and clinical approaches? The clinical method is too well known to need definition except to recall that it is essentially a bedside approach to the patient without any unnecessary restrictions. The biometric approach is more constrained by rules and regulations for obtaining reliable information, and is based on Lord Kelvin's dictum "when you can measure what you are speaking about, and express it in numbers, you know something about it; but when you cannot measure it, when you cannot express it in numbers, your knowledge is of a meager and unsatisfactory kind" (Merton, Sill, & Stigler, 1984).

Perhaps the most important distinction between the clinical and the biometric approach is in the ability of the biometrician to express the degree of certainty or uncertainty of his conclusions in some statistical form by attaching certain probabilities of being right or wrong in his judgment. While the clinician also feels degrees of uncertainty, he has no way of expressing them mathematically. Exceptional clinicians like Manfred Bleuler seem to overcome this problem.

Perhaps it is in the common objectives of clinical and biometric interviews that we can aim to bring convergence to the varying approaches. Essentially, reaching a diagnosis is the result of a series of mini-experiments in which hypotheses are tested, and further hypotheses derived based on what the patient reports, until a final diagnosis is reached. Although the open-ended interview initially may probe the specific aspects of a presenting problem in greater depth, it may also fail to detect other areas of significant pathology. The semi-structured interview provides a comprehensive and efficient overview of pathology, which may not be achieved in the open-ended format until several sessions have transpired. It is important to emphasize that these two approaches are not mutually exclusive; semi-structured interviews require the incorporation of clinical skill and judgment to recognize the nuances of patient speech and behavior that require probing.

A View of Schizophrenia in the First Half of the Century

The attitudes typical of American schools in the first half of the century towards understanding schizophrenia are typified in the personal experiences of the senior author.

> I entered the field of psychopathology serendipitously because I received my Ph.D. during the Depression in 1932 in a combined, tailor-made program at Columbia University in both experimental and educational psychology with a strong statistical bent, which I contrived despite a frown from the authorities. This was in the day before such specialties as clinical or psychometric psychology had developed. The year 1932 was a bad year to start a career—it was in the depths of the Depression. There were no jobs offered so I took a volunteer job at the New York State Psychiatric Institute (PI, as it is usually called) in the experimental psychology laboratory of the late Professor Carney Landis. Psychoanalysis was in the saddle at PI and, since the institute was established for research rather than for service, the staff selected the patients in accordance with their research program, on the basis of their suitability for psychoanalysis. My knowledge of psychopathology was rather meager and my acquaintance with psychoanalysis even less. Nevertheless, I began to apply what I had learned and began with measuring the patients' personality through specially devised personality inventories developed following Woodworth's Personal Data Sheet. These inventories were the predecessors of the MMPI. I soon discovered that the patients, though carrying the label of dementia praecox, did not behave at all like dementia praecox patients. I began to wonder whether they really fitted the textbook description. I finally mustered enough courage to discuss the matter with the Clinical Director. He looked at me sternly when I said, "I don't believe that any of these patients are dementia praecox patients, nor that they are mentally sick." His answer was: "You better believe it, or you don't belong here. They may be at an early stage in their illness, but they have it with few exceptions." I then inquired whether they would eventually deteriorate and he answered "you better believe it." This authoritative admonition stayed with me for several decades and I had only freed myself from it in the 1950s.

The tendency to diagnose schizophrenia was so strong that a mere suspicion of schizophrenia was enough to bring on the diagnosis, or as the institute director said, a touch of schizophrenia was like a touch of pregnancy. During the latter half of the 30's, somatic shock therapies—insulin and electro-convulsive therapy—were introduced, and for the first time changes in patient behavior could be observed directly without waiting years for psychotherapy to bring about its effects. Here was an open challenge to a biometrician. Could these changes be measured?

Psychological tests were of no avail since they were aimed mostly at measuring traits, which persisted, not states, which changed. Behavior rating scales were the answer and they sprouted up everywhere. Rating scales had to be produced practically overnight by such pioneers as Lorr, Wittenborn and Malamud. There is a story, probably apocryphal, told about the physiologist Hudson Hoagland, who found some biochemical change in Malamud's patients at the Worcester State Hospital and asked to see Malamud's data on the same patients. Malamud handed him his voluminous case histories. "Are there no numbers here on their behavior?" Hoagland inquired. Malamud responded, "No, but if you want numbers I'll make them up for you!" That night, with help, Malamud converted his descriptions of behavior into rating scales.

At last it became possible to see symptoms disappear or change before our very eyes. Apparently, for the first time schizophrenic behavior was seen as fleeting, not permanent or chronic, and could undergo change through intervention. Our laboratory became a watch-dog for evaluating therapies, tests, rating scales, and laboratory measures such as reaction time, flicker fusion, and psychophysiological measurement. Even the Rorschach came under scrutiny, and at that stage of its development it was found wanting as a test for identifying schizophrenia (Zubin, 1954). The conclusion was that if you treated the protocols as interview material and analyzed them for their content, the results would correlate with the content of the interviews on which the diagnoses were based. Furthermore, the determinants of movement, color, and shading were neither reliable nor valid using the scoring procedures of that period. More recently, these deficiencies have been carefully addressed by Exner and others (Exner, 1986).

The belief in the efficacy of the somatic therapies, including psychosurgery, was so strong that Stockings (1947) in England suggested that we discard our diagnostic categories entirely and classify patients according to the therapy to which they responded. Thus, those benefiting from insulin would be categorized as dysglycic, or from ECT as dysoxic. This past trend should serve as a warning against our current attempts at utilizing responses to treatment as a criterion for the diagnosis or search for subtypes. We would have to classify disorders while the therapies still worked and before they went out of vogue!

To a large extent, the development of the concept of schizophrenia reflected the place where schizophrenics were to be found—in the state hospitals. Before 1890 and the advent of Kraepelin's era, only acute cases were to be found in the rather small hospitals of the United States, where patients were brought by their families. Many of the patients were no doubt dementia praecox cases who could no longer be kept at home. The psychiatrist was merely a caretaker and not much time was available for investigations. After 1890, with the rise of immigration, the mental hospitals became overwhelmed with the aged, brain injured and chronically ill, so that they became mere warehouses for managing the patients. World War II brought a depletion of the hospital medical staffs, who were needed for the armed forces, so that state hospitals deteriorated and not much progress was seen.

However, World War II stimulated a revision of the diagnostic nomenclature because it had been based on hospitalized patients who were chronically ill, and was therefore poorly adapted to the classification of members of the armed services. There was no generally accepted national nosology. The bringing together of psychiatrists from all over the United States for the military made it necessary to develop a common language. The Veterans Administration proposed a new classification system, which did not get wide acceptance because of its bias toward the veteran population. The pressure for revision was so great that the American Psychiatric Association appointed a task force. This started the series of DSM's which went through one revision before DSM-III came on the scene.

The failure of general psychological tests as diagnostic instruments (Zubin, Eron, & Schumer, 1965) brought the realization that the only proper tool for diagnosis was the clinical interview. However, a review of the literature on the interview revealed that its reliability and validity were disastrously poor, so our group began to develop more systematic approaches. One of our friends, Mort Kramer, called attention to the discrepancy between the United States and the United Kingdom national statistics indicating that there was a 10:1 ratio of affective disorder to schizophrenia in the United Kingdom, and a converse ratio in the United States. We obtained a grant from the NIMH to study this discrepancy, and our Biometrics Research Unit utilized the newly minted systematic interviews, together with the Present State Examination of John Wing, to examine patients in metropolitan New York at the New York State Psychiatric Institute and in metropolitan London at the Maudsley Hospital. The case records in both hospitals were subsequently reviewed to determine the diagnoses according to standardized criteria.

The proportion of admissions for schizophrenia in New York, according to the hospital diagnoses, was higher than the proportion based on the revised diagnoses given by judges when standardized criteria were applied to the case histories. It is clear that the initial view of a tremendous rise in schizophrenia was not warranted by the case history analysis. When the case histories were examined for the presence of actual symptomatology, the diagnoses in the two institutions were similar. Thus, the study indicated that the discrepancy was not in the patients but in the style of applying diagnoses in the two countries (Cooper et al., 1972).

Historically, the American concept of schizophrenia has been much wider than the English concept, although before World War II it was rather narrowly defined to describe primarily hospitalized patients. When psychiatric practice extended beyond the hospital walls, the concept began to broaden as the influence of Eugen Bleuler spread and as psychoanalysis entered the picture. As milder schizophrenia began to be diagnosed it became apparent that many of the symptoms were on a continuum from mild to severe; clinicians began to see a "touch" of schizophrenia in many of their more functional patients. In this way the diagnosis of schizophrenia became diluted.

When the US-UK Project, followed by the World Health Organization study (WHO, 1979), demonstrated that the US diagnoses of schizophrenia were broader than in any other country, the need for narrowing the concept to agree with the rest of the world was recognized. Furthermore, as the results of the US-UK Project became clear, it also became apparent that these results were not merely of academic interest. Since the administration of treatment, especially drugs, was often dictated by diagnosis, many patients were given inappropriate treatment when their diagnosis was inaccurately determined. This realization introduced a careful reexamination of the efficacy of drugs. The overdiagnosis of schizophrenia in the US presented a diagnostic challenge for American psychiatrists. The four A's postulated by Eugen Bleuler, which had such a great influence in the USA (associative loosening, affective blunting, ambivalence, and autism), were not a sufficiently constraining basis for making rigorous definitions. To counter this trend, Kurt Schneider's (1959) first rank symptoms were brought to bear on diagnosis in the United Kingdom. While in retrospect these first rank symptoms may be nonspecific to schizophrenia and more useful in determining severity of the illness rather than its diagnosis, they nevertheless helped to bring about greater rigor. Thus, Bleuler's accessory symptoms were brought back into primary focus, and since these psychotic symptoms were more easily discriminated from normality with their "yes or no" presence, they added greater rigor to defining the diagnosis.

In the conference organized with the help of the American Psychopathological Association, which preceded the launching of the US-UK Project (Zubin, 1961), Carl Hempel and, somewhat earlier, Ernest Stengel, went one step further and proposed an operational approach for the definition of mental disorders by requiring that the diagnosis meet certain minimum criteria. Two more developments aided in narrowing the definition of schizophrenia. The St. Louis school at Washington University presented the first narrow set of diagnostic criteria including requirements as to the duration of symptoms (at least 6 months) and the presence of severe psychotic symptoms such as delusions and hallucinations (Feighner et al., 1972). This was soon followed by the development of the Research Diagnostic Criteria (Spitzer, Endicott, & Robins, 1978). Currently, we are awaiting the fourth version of the American Psychiatric Association's *Diagnostic and Statistical Manual* (DSM-IV) and the tenth version of the International Classification of Diseases (ICD-10).

Vulnerability Theory: A Model Integrating Disparate Etiologies

Thus far we have dealt with the phenomenology of schizophrenia as it developed in the United States with a special focus on diagnosis. Having established the reliability, if not the validity, of the diagnosis of schizophrenia, it became necessary to deal with issues of validity by examining etiology. Since there was still no known basis for etiology, a set of scientific models covering the various approaches to etiology was proposed (Zubin, 1972).

The need for scientific models to explain observed facts is well illustrated by De Sola Price in his book *Science Since Babylon* (1975). He points out that the ancient Babylonians were fact-mongers and provided sufficient data on planetary movements to be able to predict their future positions, but had no conceptual framework for their orbits. The ancient Greeks, on the other hand, were not so interested in number crunching, but were conceptually minded, so they provided the geometry for the orbit of the planets. It was not until Alexander the Great brought these two civilizations together that the modern scientific endeavor was born in which conceptual models could be tested by empirical observation. Until the 1950s, psychiatry was largely a conceptual field, in which the theories had little connection with statistics that enumerated the frequency and distribution of mental disorders.

After first suggesting that various models of etiology, (including biochemical, genetic, learning, and environmental sources), could all contribute to the etiology of schizophrenia (Zubin, 1972), it became clear that no single model was appropriate to explain all of the findings. Consequently, an integrative theoretical formulation, the Vulnerability model, was advanced (Zubin & Spring, 1977). This model postulates that an enduring vulnerability to schizophrenia results from interactions among the various contributing etiological sources, rather than from any single etiological source. The appearance of symptomatology results because the vulnerable individual fails to cope with changing stresses in the environment. Thus, vulnerability is manifested by the possession of a lower threshold for coping with stressful life events. Following the onset of symptoms, reduction of stress below threshold can be expected to lead to remission of symptoms. In essence, the theory provides a heuristic for understanding that the schizophrenic episode itself is not a permanent condition, but that the potential for episodes persists. Coincident with this interactional view of vulnerability in the development of schizophrenia are data indicating the importance of psychosocial and ecological factors, as well as data indicating less severe long-term outcomes for schizophrenic patients than had previously been claimed (Zubin, Magaziner, & Steinhauer, 1983).

The vulnerability hypothesis also predicts that indicators or markers can be found in patients prior to or following episodes, as well as among their unaffected relatives. Such familial markers, including, but not limited to, genetic factors, would reflect vulnerability, but not indicate schizophrenia per se. A framework for examining a variety of probable behavioral and neurophysiological indicators was developed (Zubin & Steinhauer, 1981). Additional developments of the vulnerability model have emphasized interactional (Nuechterlein & Dawson, 1984) or specific physiological (Mirsky & Duncan, 1986) aspects of the vulnerability dimension.

We have also been concerned with understanding how a relatively permanent vulnerability may be reconciled with a differential sensitivity to the same stressors at different points in an individual's life. Recently, we modified the basic vulnerability model by introducing a separate dimension that accounts for changes in tolerance to stress (Steinhauer et al., 1991). The tolerance dimension provides for the intervention of psychotherapeutic or biological treatments as a means of raising the individual's threshold for coping above their usual or minimal level.

Atypical Notions Regarding Schizophrenia

It is clear that we share common ground with Manfred Bleuler in that our views of schizophrenia are not the same as those of our respective cultures. We differ from the traditional views of schizophrenia with regard to the following notions:

1.   A more optimistic view of outcome. A disbelief that once schizophrenic, always schizophrenic, i.e., that it is not a permanently chronic condition necessarily leading to deterioration.

2.   An acceptance of vulnerability, and not chronicity, as the permanent characteristic of schizophrenia.

3.   An acceptance of the belief that schizophrenia is an episodic disorder. Not only is this a consequence of the view necessitated by the vulnerability hypothesis, it is also born out in reviewing a variety of long-term follow-up studies (Zubin et al., 1983), including the work of Manfred Bleuler.

However, some of our deviations from establishment thinking may not be fully shared by Professor Bleuler.

Kraepelin was probably wrong in endowing the schizophrenic with an intact sensorium. During the past three decades quite a number of brain function indicators have been identified that discriminate between schizophrenics and general population control groups, if not between schizophrenics and other mentally disordered individuals. Examples of such indicators include: the amplitudes of the P300 component of the event-related potential; pupillary dilation response; heart rate changes related to information processing activities; smooth pursuit eye movement abnormalities; behavioral indicators of vigilance (e.g., the continuous performance test); and iconic memory (e.g., span of attention).

Perhaps the most convincing evidence that the brain of the schizophrenic is not intact comes from the comparison of the brain structures of discordant identical twin pairs. The presence of greater ventricular enlargement in the brain of the affected twin compared to that of the unaffected twin (Suddath et al., 1990) seems to imply that the brain of the schizophrenic, and presumably the sensorium, are not intact. Although it is not yet certain whether the observed changes are antecedents or consequences (including possible consequences of treatment), the results do offer a potential testimony for the environmental triggering of a genetic vulnerability. Further evidence of environmental triggering is provided by Tienari's findings that the schizophrenic phenotype emerges primarily in those vulnerable adoptees who are subjected to a disruptive family environment, and not in the equally vulnerable adoptees whose families are not disruptive (Tienari et al., 1978).

Kraepelin may also have erred in his significant clinical contribution regarding the absolute separation of dementia praecox (schizophrenia) from manic depressive psychosis. Although it has served heuristically to stimulate investigations, this separation has not been confirmed. While the excess of schizophrenic, but not manic depressive, illness in the biological relatives of schizophrenic adoptees offers some evidence for specific genetic transmission of these functional disorders, the presence of the manic depressives still has to be explained. The difficulty for the dichotomous scheme is easily seen in the diagnostic dilemma produced by atypical or intermediate cases, a dilemma that has often been resolved through the arbitrary imposition of a single diagnosis. To resolve this issue will require developing models that will distinguish, on the one hand, a single vulnerability with variable expression, and on the other hand, two independent vulnerabilities coexisting in the same individual, perhaps due to assortative mating (as suggested by Dr. Loring Ingraham, personal communication). It may be that the two functional disorders form a continuous spectrum with many intermediate types, rather than a dichotomy, so that what we have is a psychotic manifestation that can assume either a schizophrenic or an affective expression depending on premorbid personality, local traditions, ecological niche, social network, and timing of environmental trauma.

Furthermore, Brockington (1988) argues that Kraepelin's formulation of dementia praecox lacks the essential characteristics which Aristotle demanded of a category—a single essence for identifying the concept. Instead, he notes three essences or defining principles highlighted by Kraepelin: a convergence to a defect state, the schizm [sic] or fission within the psyche, and the autistic absorption with a private world. "These principles are all completely different, and thus the richness of the psychopathology of schizophrenia, which Kraepelin and Bleuler described so vividly and which gives the 'disease' its fascination and appeal, is its greatest weakness, denying any possibility of bringing the concept to a clear focus" (Brockington, 1988, p. 6). It is possible that the three Kraepelinian essences may eventually be traceable to a unique central nervous system and/or genetic deviation.

As for the effect of the biometric approach on the problem of schizophrenic essence, the formulations of DSM-III and the RDC disclaim anything but sheer atheoretical empiricism. As a result, as Brockington, Kendell, and Leff (1978) remark, "the previous state of inarticulate confusion in the diagnosis of schizophrenia has been replaced by a 'babble' of precise but differing formulations of the same concept." The consequence has been a proliferation of interviews, diagnostic criteria, and nosologies; it is now time to reconcile the data from these various approaches.

Finally, we suggest that attention be paid to the self-healing capacities of the individual. We do not yet know the reasons that some patients appear to outgrow their disorder after a decade or so, or understand why some patients suddenly cease to exhibit symptoms. Much of this may reflect the tendency of the organism to heal itself. Interventions should be aimed at helping the self-healing process to occur. Moreover, greater attention should be paid to what behaviors and attitudes the patient brings to the healing process. John Strauss has pointed out that we rarely ask the patients what they are doing to help themselves, and this is certainly a notion that should be pursued.

Why the establishment disagrees with us with regard to optimistic outcome is an interesting question. In the following quote, Manfred Bleuler explains his father's pessimism about schizophrenia:

> From 1886 to 1889, E. Bleuler dedicated himself completely to his community of schizophrenics as director of the remote psychiatric clinic of Rheinau, which was then an isolated, rural sector of Switzerland. Two decades later, during and after the First World War, he went back to Rheinau to visit about once a year, usually when the weather was fine during the summer. His former schizophrenic patients always greeted him warmly, enthusiastically. Much as these greetings pleased him, he usually made the painful observation, "Most of them did seem to have deteriorated." Then, depressed, he would ask, "Is there really nothing that can stop this disease?" But E. Bleuler did not know how many improved patients were out for their Sunday walks during his visits, and certainly not how many had been released and were living at home, recovered. Had he known, and if he had not continued to meet only the most severe cases among his old problem children, his assessment of schizophrenia would have been strongly influenced. A number of generations of clinical psychiatrists had experiences similar to his (M. Bleuler, 1978, p. 413).

We try to explain the pessimism in the USA by two factors. First, there has been a persistence of the degeneration theory developed in the middle of the nineteenth century, which presumed that the first generation developed neurosis, the second generation developed mental retardation and mental disorder, and the third generation finally disappeared for lack of propagation, only to be replaced by newcomers in subhuman development. Though science, especially genetics, has long ago disposed of this theory, it still persists in the zeitgeist and is at the bottom of the stigma that is still attached to the families of schizophrenics. It also persists in the Kraepelinian heritage of the expectation of deterioration even though Kraepelin himself had disavowed the theory in his later years.

Second, there is the experience from the daily workload of most clinicians, who deal primarily with recidivist patients who either relapse or remain chronic, and thus provides a biased view of the outcome of schizophrenia. Like Eugen Bleuler, they forget about the patients who never return because they no longer need treatment.

Future Directions for Clinical Investigation

The bulk of the 30 or 40 billion dollars spent on schizophrenia annually is spent on relapsing or chronic cases. If we could nick the relapse rate by only 10%, it would save billions of dollars, many times the total research budget allotted to schizophrenia. In surveying the literature, one notices that relapse appears far from being an indigenous characteristic of schizophrenia. From 23 to 50% of schizophrenics never relapse after their first episode. The WHO (1979) cross-cultural studies find 35% non-relapsers in developing countries and 19% in developed countries, while Luc Ciompi in Bern, Switzerland, reports 10% in his studies (Ciompi, 1980). With our currently reliable diagnostic methods we ought to be able to contrast patients who are similar diagnostically in their first episode and then determine what factors differentiate those who later relapse from those who do not.

We will conclude with an aphorism that characterizes the essence of the difference between the optimists' and the pessimists' views of schizophrenia. The philosophical optimist suggests that this is the best of all possible worlds, to which the pessimist responds "I'm afraid so." The pessimists, who are adherents of the chronic disease model, believe that the schizophrenic, for the most part, is a continuously sick person who once in awhile relapses into health. The optimists, who are adherents of the vulnerability model, believe that the schizophrenic, for the most part, is essentially a healthy person who possesses a continuing vulnerability, and who once in awhile suffers an episode of illness. We obviously embrace the latter view.

References

Bleuler, M. (1978). *The schizophrenic disorders: Long-term patient and family studies.* Translated by S.M. Clemens. New Haven, CT: Yale University Press.

Brockington, I.F. (1988). A critical view of the concept of schizophrenia. In: Williams, R., & Dalby, J.T. (Ed.), *Depression in schizophrenia.* New York: Plenum Press, pp. 5-12.

Brockington, I.F., Kendell, R.E., & Leff, J.P. (1978). Definitions of schizophrenia: Concordance and prediction of outcome. *Psychological Medicine, 7,* 387-398.

Ciompi, L. (1980). The natural history of schizophrenia in the long term. *British Journal of Psychiatry, 136,* 413-420.

Cooper, J.E., Kendall, R.E., Gurland, B.J., Sharpe, L., Copeland, J.R.M., & Simon, R. (1972). *Psychiatric diagnosis in New York and London: A comparative study of mental hospital admissions.* Maudsley Monograph. London: Oxford University.

Exner, J.E. (1986). *The Rorschach: A comprehensive system. Volume 1: Basic foundations (2nd edition).* New York: Wiley & Sons.

Feighner, J.P., Robins, E., Guze, S.B., Woodruff, R.A., Winokur, G., & Munoz, R. (1972). Diagnostic criteria for use in psychiatric research. *Archives of General Psychiatry, 26,* 57-63.

Huxley, J.S. (1940). Introductory: Towards the new systematics. In: Huxley, J.S. (Ed.), *The New Systematics.* Oxford: Clarendon Press.

Merton, R.K., Sill, D., & Stigler, M. (1984). The Kelvin dictum and social science: An excursion into the history of an idea. *Journal of the History of the Behavioral Sciences, 20,* 319-331.

Mirsky A.F. & Duncan C.C. (1986). Etiology and expression of schizophrenia: Neurobiological and psychosocial factors. *Annual Review of Psychology, 37,* 291-319.

Nuechterlein, K.H. & Dawson, M.E. (1984). A heuristic vulnerability/stress model of schizophrenic episodes. *Schizophrenia Bulletin, 10,* 300-312.

Price, D.J. de Solla (1975). *Science Since Babylon,* Enl. ed. New Haven, CT: Yale University Press.

Schneider, K. (1959). *Clinical Psychopathology.* English translation by M.W. Hamilton and E.W. Anderson, 89-114. New York: Grune & Stratton.

Spitzer, R.L., Endicott, J., & Robins, E. (9178). Research Diagnostic Criteria: Rationale and reliability. *Archives of General Psychiatry, 35,* 773-782.

Steinhauer, S.R., Zubin, J., Condray, R., Shaw, D.B., Peters, J.L., & van Kammen, D.P. (1991). Electrophysiological and behavioral signs of attentional disturbance in schizophrenics and their siblings. In: Tamminga, C.A., and Schulz, S.C. (Eds.), *Schizophrenia research. Advances in neuropsychiatry and psychopharmacology, vol. 1.* New York: Raven Press, pp. 169-178.

Stockings, G. (1947). *The metabolic brain diseases and their treatment.* Baltimore: Williams & Wilkins.

Suddath, R.L., Christison, G.W., Torrey, E.F., Casanova, M.F., & Weinberger, D.R. (1990). Anatomical abnormalities in the brains of monozygotic twins discordant for schizophrenia. *The New England Journal of Medicine, 322,* 789-794.

Tienari, P., Sorri, A., Lahti, I., Naarala, M., Wahlberg, K.-E., Moring, J., Pohjola, J., & Wynne, L.C. (1978). Genetic and psychosocial factors in schizophrenia: The Finnish adoptive family study. *Schizophrenia Bulletin, 13,* 477-484.

World Health Organization (1979). *Schizophrenia -- An International Follow-up Study.* New York: John Wiley & Sons.

Zubin, J. (1954). Failures of the Rorschach technique. *Journal of Projective Techniques, 18,* 303-315.

Zubin, J. (Ed.) (1961). *Field studies in the mental disorders.* New York: Grune & Stratton.

Zubin, J. (1972). Scientific models for psychopathology in the 1970's. *Seminars in Psychiatry, 4*, 283-296.

Zubin, J., Eron, L., & Schumer, F. (1965). *An experimental approach to projective techniques.* New York: Wiley.

Zubin, J., Magaziner, J., and Steinhauer, S.R. (1983). The metamorphosis of schizophrenia: From chronicity to vulnerability. *Psychological Medicine, 13*, 551-571.

Zubin J. & Spring, B. (1977). Vulnerability: A new view of schizophrenia. *Journal of Abnormal Psychology, 86*, 103-126.

Zubin, J. & Steinhauer, S.R. (1981). How to break the logjam in schizophrenia: A look beyond genetics. *The Journal of Nervous and Mental Disease, 169*, 477-492.

3
Autism: Core of the Schizophrenic Reaction

Erik Strömgren

Introduction

The question in the title of this book can be answered in different ways. It may be understood as aiming at some definition, maybe obtained by a consensus, circumscribing a group of individuals who can be said to belong to a special class, defined by means of clear criteria that should enable everybody working clinically with schizophrenics to know fairly exactly what kind of individual is meant by the definition. Such a consensus would, however, still not tell us what schizophrenia really is. The definition would probably say nothing about the causes and development of the disorder. The consensus definition would just work as a tool for understanding among those who work with schizophrenics, some of whom would, however, regard the definition as being too broad, and others as being too narrow. At the present state of our knowledge of the causes of schizophrenia viewpoints concerning etiology differ greatly.

Background

The different ways of looking at schizophrenia depend very much on the kind of experience the individual researcher has had with schizophrenics. Some have seen a great number of schizophrenics during a long period, and have seen many different clinical forms and courses. Others may have seen relatively few schizophrenics but may have obtained an intimate knowledge about just these patients. Still others may have no real experience with schizophrenics but have been fascinated by what others have told them about schizophrenia and may have felt inclined to try to understand what the process is really about.

It is my feeling that it would be advisable that anybody who takes part in this important discussion should state which kinds of experience he or she has had with schizophrenics, and, if possible which other disorders he or she has encountered for comparison with schizophrenia. Following this suggestion I shall just briefly give information about my own background for talking about schizophrenia.

I started reading Freud and Eugen Bleuler quite early and became deeply impressed especially by Bleuler's writings about schizophrenia. As a student I obtained my first contact with schizophrenics in different psychiatric wards, working with acute as well as chronic schizophrenics. Since then I have spent most of my time working with psychiatric patients, and estimate that I have met about 3000 schizophrenics, having close contact with quite a fraction of them, more superficial contact with the rest.

Possibilities for Definitions

Before a definition of the concept of schizophrenia is attempted, it is necessary to state in which different senses the word schizophrenia can be used. There are three possibilities. The term can be used nosologically, symptomatologically, or syndromatologically.

The *nosological* variant supposes that such a thing as a schizophrenic disease really exists, in the sense that a specific etiology causes a recognizable disease process which again gives a certain number of symptoms.

The *symptomatological* variant, on the other hand, only requires that certain types of symptoms are present, some of which may be regarded as more or less necessary for the diagnosis.

Finally, the diagnosis of schizophrenia can be regarded as dependent on the presence of certain *syndromes*, symptom clusters. Neither the symptomatological nor the syndromatological definition supposes that there should be a specific etiology behind the symptoms or the syndromes. The nosological definition, on the other hand, does not demand that any symptoms should be specific, not to say obligatory.

The syndromatological viewpoint has also manifested itself in the concept of *reaction types*. A schizophrenic reaction type should consist of a certain combination of symptoms, which could appear as reactions to many different kinds of etiologies, which may be organic as well as psychological, or combinations of the two. One extreme would be the schizophrenialike states occurring during the course of Huntington's chorea. Another extreme the sensitive delusion of reference described so vividly by Ernst Kretschmer, occurring as understandable reactions to specific kinds of mental stress.

Now a brief view of the *history* of the concept of schizophrenia. It is well known that around the middle of the nineteenth century many psychiatrists were in favor of the "unitary psychosis," the *"Einheitspsychose"* as prominent German psychiatrists (Zeller, Griesinger) called it. It was felt that although symptoms and course might differ widely in psychotic disorders, they were in fact just the expressions of one singular disease which could take any form and any course. Gradually, however, it became increasingly clear that certain disorders could be singled out which had an obvious organic background; for instance, syphilitic general paresis, senile dementia, and a number of others. However, in the majority of psychoses it was not possible to demonstrate an organic origin although in most cases it was supposed that they were of a hereditary nature. Kraepelin was responsible for a decisive clarification during the 1890s when he demonstrated, through huge empirical studies on the symptomatology and course of the so-called endogenous disorders, that there were high correlations between symptoms and course. This enabled him to establish a *dichotomy*, to distinguish dementia praecox from manic depressive disorder. This observation was of immense importance both for practical and for theoretical reasons. For the patients and their relatives it was, of course, essential to know as much as possible about the prognosis of a mental disorder, and for psychiatric research it seemed to be of basic importance that there was a possibility that these disorders also differed with regard to etiology.

On the other hand, even if the two disorders were now demonstrated to be clinically different, they had two important features in common: there was no demonstrable organic disorder present in the patients' brains, and in the clinical picture there were no symptoms present of the kinds usually seen in organic brain disorder. However, this did not restrain Kraepelin from believing that both disorders were due to underlying organic disorders.

When Eugen Bleuler introduced the term schizophrenia in 1908, he did not intend to create a new concept; he just wanted to suggest a new term for the concept of dementia praecox. He found the term inadequate because these patients were not "demented," their intellectual faculties seemed in most cases unimpaired; further, the disease did not always start "praecociter," i.e., in youth. The term *schizophrenia* (splitting of mind), on the other hand, pointed to fundamental features of the symptomatology. Bleuler did not regard schizophrenia as a nosological entity; several pathogenic agents might lead to the same clinical picture. Bleuler, like Kraepelin, regarded the etiology of schizophrenia as organic but he did not interpret all schizophrenic symptoms as direct consequences of the underlying organic process; he distinguished between "basic" symptoms and "accessory" symptoms, respectively (the terms "primary" and "secondary" symptoms have also been used), the basic symptoms being caused directly by the organic brain process, namely: disturbances of the association processes and emotional reactions and "autistic" disturbances of contact with other human beings. All other symptoms—delusions, hallucinations, catatonic symptoms, etc.—he regarded as psychologically understandable reactions to the presence of the basic symptoms. The distinction between basic and accessory symptoms was strengthened by the observation that the basic symptoms never disappeared, while accessory symptoms were often subject to change and might disappear intermittently or permanently. Bleuler (1911) and his associate Jung (1907) showed convincingly how many of the schizophrenic symptoms could be interpreted in terms of psychoanalytic concepts. Jung also regarded schizophrenia as the consequence of an organic brain process.

In the overall clinical picture, the accessory, psychologically determined symptoms could be quite dominant; they were, in principle, reversible. This was an explanation for the fact that in many schizophrenics sooner or later, gradually or suddenly, the great majority of symptoms might disappear leaving only some of the basic symptoms. Bleuler's delimitation of schizophrenia was very similar to Kraepelin's delimitation of dementia praecox, but he added descriptions of some mild cases of schizophrenia that Kraepelin would probably not have included in his concept. Both investigators stressed the poor prognosis of the disorder, although in a small percentage recovery seemed to occur.

Symptoms of Schizophrenia

Since the etiology of schizophrenia is still largely unknown, any attempt at defining schizophrenia will have to rely on symptoms and, perhaps, course. An accurate description of the symptoms which are regarded as relevant is therefore the first step on the road to definition.

It was immanent in Bleuler's new terminology that "splitting" should be a basic trait, primarily a splitting of the associations that did not seem to follow comprehensible ways; but also a splitting between ideas and emotions, ideas often not being accompanied by adequate affects. With regard to two other important symptoms, autism and ambivalence, the interpretation had to be qualified. Although autism was a very characteristic symptom in schizophrenics, Bleuler regarded some degree of autism as occurring also within normal psychology, the difference between normal and pathological autism consisting in the fact that the latter was fixed, and the former, to a certain degree, flexible. Unfortunately, the term autism has been the cause of much confusion over the years, some psychiatrists regarding autism as a pathognomonic symptom in schizophrenia, others as a more or less normal feature. The peak of confusion was reached when Kanner coined a rare disease occurring in infants as "infantile autism," in spite of the fact that this disorder, which should rightly be called Kanner's disorder, has nothing to do with schizophrenia.

The concept of ambivalence comprises similar problems. It is obvious that ambivalence occurs in all human beings and also that it is a very prominent symptom in schizophrenics, the difference between groups being primarily temporal; ambivalence in non-schizophrenics usually shows itself in an oscillation between one viewpoint and its opposite, whereas in schizophrenics the two components may be present and active simultaneously.

Disturbances of self are the most characteristic of schizophrenic symptoms; the feeling of changes in one's own personality, internal splitting, lack of command of thoughts and feelings, the feeling that others take command of one's acts and thoughts, that thoughts are taken away, and that other alien thoughts are inserted.

Delusions occur in all schizophrenics but very often are not of a nature which can be said to be specific to schizophrenia. The same applies to hallucinations. It is, however, certain that in schizophrenics these may be of the same intensity as real sensory experiences.

Much research has concentrated on cognitive functions in schizophrenics. Different kinds of disturbances have been ascertained but none of these are seen in *all* schizophrenics. Their relevance for the diagnosis is doubtful and, in any case, it can safely be stated that a true "dementia" of the type that occurs in chronic organic brain disorders does not develop in schizophrenia.

One more feature is crucial: all the symptoms mentioned are of no relevance for the diagnosis of schizophrenia if there is a simultaneous disturbance of consciousness in the patient. The symptoms are only important for the diagnosis if there is clarity of consciousness. On the other hand, if several of the symptoms mentioned are present in a patient in a state of clear consciousness, a diagnosis of schizophrenia is highly probable. The next question is then: can we relate these groups of symptoms to any *nosological entity* which can be regarded as the basis for the symptoms? If research has not yet taught us very much about the etiology of schizophrenia, it has at least made it highly probable that in a nosological sense schizophrenia is heterogeneous. Bleuler talked about a "group of schizophrenias." Research has taught us that, in the etiology, both genetic and environmental factors are involved. From twin studies we know that only about 45% of the causation can be of genetic nature—the environment is responsible for the major part. No specific exogenous factors have, however, as yet been ascertained. It is probable that several external factors can contribute to the origin of a schizophrenic development.

The genetic background seems to be heterogeneous as well. According to recent research a major gene may be responsible for some cases of schizophrenia but certainly not for all. It is not even certain that the genes responsible can be regarded, in a strict sense, as pathological. Manfred Bleuler has mentioned the possibility that the hereditary background may not consist in the presence of abnormal genes but in an unfortunate combination of normal genes. Other researchers have talked about multifactorial inheritance, in the sense that the genetic backgrounds of schizophrenia and normality may be characterized as continua, and that threshold mechanisms are responsible for the development of the schizophrenic process.

As mentioned, the environmental factors may also be very heterogeneous. At present, nobody knows whether they are more of an organic or psychological nature; even within these two groups there may be heterogeneity.

With regard to signs and symptoms of organic lesions in schizophrenics, a great number of publications have appeared in recent years. Although there is evidence that such features occur in some schizophrenics, none of them occur in all or even in the majority of schizophrenics. Their importance for the schizophrenic disorder is, therefore, still quite obscure.

In this connection I would like to make a comment on an important section in Professor Sarbin's contribution to this book. Quoting an unpublished paper by M. Boyle, "Is schizophrenia what it was? A reanalysis of Kraepelin's and Bleuler's population," he discusses the interesting problem of the disappearance of catatonic symptomatology in schizophrenics during the last half century. Boyle has come to the conclusion that what Kraepelin and Bleuler described as catatonic schizophrenia was not schizophrenia but simply post-encephalitic parkinsonism. This is, indeed, a bold statement which can only arise on the basis of a deep ignorance of neurological evidence. To any experienced clinician, there is a fundamental difference between catatonic symptoms and parkinsonism. The motor symptoms in the two disorders show fundamental differences. In addition, in patients with post-encephalitic parkinsonism there are conspicuous changes in the spinal fluid which do not occur in schizophrenics. In parkinsonism there are specific cellular changes in certain regions of the brain—none of these are present in schizophrenia. Needless to say, both Kraepelin and Bleuler were familiar with both disorders and could distinguish between them, as clearly displayed in their textbooks.

The disappearance of catatonia has a quite different explanation: it took place gradually after the introduction of shock therapies and especially pharmacological therapies. Unfortunately, the disappearance of some of the most conspicuous symptoms in schizophrenia did not imply that schizophrenia was cured in these patients. We know that great changes can occur in the clinical picture of schizophrenia in connection with both somatic and psychological therapies and also in connection with non-therapeutic events. The following case histories illustrate how spectacular changes in the clinical picture can exist without a change of the fundamental schizophrenic symptoms.

One of Eugen Bleuler's patients was a middle-aged woman who had been severely schizophrenic for several years, disturbed, violent, and uncooperative. She had to be kept permanently in a disturbed ward. One day a fire broke out in the ward and all patients had to be transferred to a different ward. The patient changed her behavior completely, became sensible and cooperative, and she remained so. When she was asked how it was possible that she could be so different now from how she used to be, her reply was: "I do not want to be taken back to the ward where they burn the patients," indicating that her delusional inner life had not basically changed.

One of my own patients, a 39-year-old farmer's wife, was admitted to a psychiatric hospital in a severe catatonic state which continued for the next 3½ years. She was profoundly disturbed, with hallucinations and delusions, catatonic hyperkinesia, and deep autism. This was before the era of active psychiatric therapy, and nothing could be done to change her state. One day a message came that her husband had fallen down from the roof of the barn and broken both legs. The patient responded to this message by getting out of her bed, saying that now of course she had to go home to take care of everything there. She discussed these matters in such a reasonable, matter-of-fact way that she was discharged immediately—and never admitted again. Four years later I had a talk with her husband, who informed me that she was still well. She was not exactly the same as she had been before the disease; she was now a little absent-minded and difficult to contact. But there were no overt symptoms of schizophrenia, no signs of hallucinations or delusions. She was an efficient housewife. Ten years after her discharge, I happened to meet her when she was admitted to a neurological ward in which I was working. She was still a little absent-minded, and emotional contact with her was difficult to obtain. But nobody in the ward had any suspicion that she was mentally ill. Here psychological factors had obviously been able to relieve the patient of all schizophrenic symptoms except a mild degree of autism.

A number of years ago when I started working in the Aarhus Psychiatric Hospital, I soon got acquainted with a nice, middle-aged man who worked in the administration office. He was known as a most conscientious worker, very quiet, reticent, but always attentive in discussions concerning his work. I learned that in fact he was a patient who had been in the hospital for many years. The first years after his admission were dominated by paranoid symptomatology. After this followed a catatonic period which lasted for seven years. During this period he would stand up all the time, doing nothing. In the evening he had to be put to bed by force; during the day, he would stand in the same spot, completely inactive; he gradually developed oedema of his feet and legs. One day this state changed suddenly. He was transferred to an open ward and stayed there until his discharge several years later; his conduct was now completely normal. He started to work in the office in a very efficient way. In conversations with doctors, however, he still revealed some delusions.

In fact, nobody knew of any factors that might have caused his deterioration or his improvement. It was tempting to ask him, in spite of the well known fact that schizophrenics very often do not answer such questions (because they regard the answer to be so obvious that only a silly person would ask). I thought, however, that being a newcomer I had a right to be uninformed about things that had happened before I came, so one day I just asked him why he had been standing up for seven years, doing nothing. He looked a little astonished, but soon realized that of course I could not know, and then he readily explained what had happened. One day the head nurse had passed by him, uttering a remark that seemed to him to be a hint that she found him to be lazy. As he felt that he was in no way lazy, he was extremely hurt by this, and decided to demonstrate that he was certainly not lazy: "And I can assure you, doctor, that there is nothing as exhausting as standing up for years." Obviously he thought that his standing up all the time was the best way in which he could demonstrate that he was not lazy. My next question was why he had ceased standing upright. The explanation was quite simple: one day a new doctor made a round in the disturbed ward where this patient had been for years, and decided that the patient should be transferred to a different ward. As this second ward was a place in which all patients were engaged in useful work, the patient immediately "understood" that his transfer to that ward was proof that he was now regarded as a good worker. Therefore he could stop his demonstration immediately.

The last two cases demonstrate how long-lasting, completely incapacitating catatonic symptoms can both originate and again cease as a consequence of delusional misinterpretations of facts. The third case history, by the way, also illustrates how difficult it can be to make the distinction, so popular in recent years, between "negative" and "positive" symptoms in schizophrenia. Is it a negative symptom to stand up for seven years? Some would perhaps say yes. Others would regard it as a unique positive accomplishment.

One intriguing observation must affect the reasoning concerning etiology, namely, that schizophrenia seems to have the same incidence in all populations in which it has been studied (Sartorius et al., 1986). If this contention holds true, a great number of environmental factors can be ruled out as etiological components in schizophrenia: social factors, nutritional factors, general health condition, etc.; factors which vary so widely among populations that, if they were of any etiological importance for schizophrenia, they must necessarily cause great diversity in the incidence of the disorder. Etiological environmental factors may instead be common to all human societies. The pathogenic experiences must occur very early in life, before the environmental situation begins to differ according to the respective cultural circumstances.

We may be left with a description of the development of schizo-phrenic disorders which implies that schizophrenic symptomatology is a *reaction type* that can be elicited by a number of different causative factors. There may be a *vulnerability* which is more or less genetically determined, but also affected by early environmental agents; later, different precipitating factors of a more or less specific nature may release a schizophrenic process.

This description seems quite reasonable, but it still is only a model for which we have little evidence. So it seems that we are left with only the possibility of describing a number of symptoms and syndromes that are more or less specific to the group of patients that we are inclined to call schizophrenic. We may now ask which of these symptoms or syndromes should be regarded as being especially relevant for the diagnosis. Are any of them specific, or even pathognomonic? Much attention has been paid to some of the symptomatological criteria described by Kurt Schneider as being essential for the diagnosis of schizophrenia, symptoms which he considered as belonging to the "first rank." Schneider found that these symptoms had turned out to be of special importance when psychiatrists made a diagnosis of schizophrenia. First-rank symptoms include the following: the patient hearing his own thoughts spoken aloud; hearing voices talking to each other about the patient; hearing voices that comment on the patient's behavior; feelings of the patient's body being influenced by outside forces; feelings of thoughts being removed or foreign thoughts being inserted into the mind; feeling that thoughts are broadcast to other people; feeling that emotions, drives, and intentions are dictated by external forces. Schneider concluded: "When it is stated that a patient has such experiences, and there is no evidence of a physical disorder, we in all modesty are talking about schizophrenia."

Most psychiatrists will agree that this selection of symptoms is of great relevance for the diagnosis of schizophrenia, but empirical studies have shown that they are, nevertheless, not specific, and that at least some of them are not present at all in some schizophrenics; paranoid schizophrenics may have very few of them.

It is, by the way, quite interesting that Schneider stressed that there should be "no evidence of a physical disorder" in spite of the fact that he regarded schizophrenia as a psychosis, and that he only found it permissible to use the term psychosis for disorders that were physically determined.

The crucial question now is whether any of these symptoms—or any other symptoms—can be said to be specific, or even pathognomonic, for schizophrenia. Manfred Bleuler, on the basis of his long-standing and intensive personal studies on schizophrenics, seems to have come to the conclusion that the presence of autism is the most important and most relevant criterion for the diagnosis of schizophrenic disorders. I tend to agree with him. The next question then is whether we can give a sufficiently accurate description of the symptom of autism. This is, unfortunately, difficult. But we can at least make some negative statements. Autism has nothing to do with the form of dementia that we see in organic brain disorder. Autism does not affect any of the intellectual processes. It is a disturbance of emotional contact with other human beings, but is basically different from what is called autism in children with Kanner's syndrome. If you talk with adult Kanner's patients who are sufficiently intellectually intact, they can assure you that they do want emotional contact with other humans. The problem, they say, is that when they are occupied by a special interest they feel intrusion by other people as most disturbing and painful, especially when others try to distract them from what they are concentrating on. The situation is different for schizophrenics. In many situations it seems as if they are simply unconsciously afraid of establishing contact with other humans, maybe for fear of loosing this contact again, a fear which probably has arisen as a reaction to catastrophic emotional experiences in early childhood.

It seems to be a very important task for psychopathologists to try to understand and describe schizophrenic autism in such a way that it may become easier to ascertain the presence of autism, this mechanism that may be of pathognomonic importance in schizophrenia.

Unfortunately, a description of autism is usually impossible to obtain from the patients themselves. The symptoms are so basic and so subjective that schizophrenics cannot give an objective description of it. Exceptions do, however, occur.

A 35-year-old woman had been schizophrenic since she was 16 and over the years had displayed all kinds of schizophrenic symptoms, including some of the most severe ones. She was very intelligent and was eager to explain her inner life. She had read psychiatric textbooks and could see clearly that psychiatrists must necessarily regard her as schizophrenic. She gave me special information about the schizophrenic person's experience of autism and mental splitting. With regard to autism she stressed that schizophrenics have very special thoughts about themselves. In addition, schizophrenics are supersensitive to a terrible degree. More specifically, they cannot tolerate being judged and evaluated in an incorrect way. Once she said to me:

> For me it is so that when I am in a group and one of the others says something which shows that this person has totally misjudged me, then suddenly I cannot at all hear what that person is saying. I can hear what the others say, but not what that person is saying.

The patient thus experiences autism as a defense mechanism which is enormously efficient for her. She also stresses that of course she is willing to contribute to the understanding of schizophrenic mechanisms, but that this is very painful for her because then she must talk about things which she definitely would not like to think of. What makes it possible for her, nevertheless, to give a description is that she has a special motivation; namely, the hope that the exposition of the schizophrenic mechanisms can have the consequence that she and other schizophrenics will be treated with greater understanding. It is obvious that this exposition is very stressful for her, and it is also clear that a schizophrenic who does not have a similar motivation will find it much easier to escape into autism behind which their phantasies can flourish.

In summary I can say that I regard schizophrenia as a reaction form, which has a heterogeneous etiological background. In most cases there is a genetic predisposition which may be monogenic, or multifactorial, or both; organic hazards to the brain may increase the vulnerability. The environmental enhancing factors may be of a physical or a psychological nature. But the core of the schizophrenic reaction form is autism, which is a defense mechanism that is applied when the person experiences intolerable idiosyncratic situations.

Having said this, I feel that I have already said far too much. Definitions are dangerous; they may conceal or even twist the facts as some popular diagnostic systems in fact do. I have once said—and I would like to repeat it quite emphatically: until we know better, a certain amount of obscurity may be much more useful than brilliant pseudo-clarity.

The psychopathological explanation of autism does not in any way preclude the possibility that many different agents, genetic or environmental, may increase the vulnerability to the psychological developments which are essential for schizophrenia.

References

Bleuler, E. (1908). Die prognose der dementia praecox (schizophreniegruppe). *Allg. Zeitschr. f. Psychiatrie u. Psychisch-Gerichtliche Medizin, 65*, 435-464.

Bleuler, E. (1911). Dementia praecox oder die gruppe der schizophrenien. In G. Aschaffenburg (Ed.), *Handbuch der Psychiatrie*. Leipzig: Deuticke.

Bleuler, M. (1972). *Die schizophrenen geistesstörungen.* Stuttgart: Georg Thieme Verlag.

Jung, C.G. (1907). *Über die psychologie der dementia praecox.* Halle/Saale: Marhold.

Sartorius, N., Jablensky, A., Korten, A., Ernberg, G., Anker, M., Cooper, J.E., & Day, R. (1986). Early manifestations and first-contact incidence of schizophrenia in different cultures. *Psychological Medicine, 16*, 909-928.

Schneider, K. (1966). *Klinische psychopathologie, 7. Ausgabe.* Stuttgart: Georg Thieme Verlag.

4

Schizophrenia Is a Word

Rue L. Cromwell

Schizophrenia is a word, no more, no less. It has some of the same benefits given us by other elements in our language and communication, including the scientific sort; but it also has some of the same vulnerabilities and shortcomings.

We do not know when man first invented language. We do know that by at least two million years ago our forebears had invented concepts. We know this from the fact that our forebears had by this time invented tools. When a tool is made in one stimulus environment to be used at another time in a different stimulus environment for a specified purpose, there can be no doubt that the tool maker is a concept-bearing organism. Concepts themselves are tools, and it can be argued that the capacity of our ancestors to develop concepts was more important to their survival and evolution than the specific artifactual tools that have been found would suggest.

It is likely that language also developed about this time. George Herbert Mead (1934) presented three criteria for the origin of language. First, a response is made by the sender (the symbol). Second, a response is made by the receiver (the meaning or referent). Third, the behavior (or its medium) must be transportable to another time and situation.

Even now, language and communication have their limits. I am reminded of a colleague who was interviewing a candidate for a faculty position at an academic institution for the deaf. The candidate was deaf. My colleague has only one arm. While driving the candidate from one meeting site to another, my colleague was having difficulty signing and managing the steering wheel at the same time. So, he asked the candidate if he would hold the steering wheel while he gave an extended message in sign language. The candidate obliged. Then, both discovered that if the candidate managed the steering wheel he would also have to keep his eyes on the road rather than on the signing.

So, Mead's criterion of transportability has its limits. To transport a word such as schizophrenia to another culture likewise has its transportability difficulties if the boundaries of reported sensation and ideation are different.

But the foregoing is not the reason why I introduce Mead's criteria. Two other reasons are more salient. First, Mead's criteria make clear that language is arbitrary. The word and the concept of schizophrenia are, therefore, arbitrary. Second, words, especially their meanings, are heavily dependent upon their receivers (listeners, users). No matter what the initial intent of the sender, this is the case. No matter what we should conclude or prescribe in these chapters, the meaning ascribed to the term schizophrenia will ultimately be determined by those who use it. The use of this term is not, of course, restricted to professional or scientific users.

With the turn of this century rules came to be made about the use of words in science (e.g., see Bergmann & Spence, 1941). Contemporary with Freud in Vienna, although with no known inter-communication, the Vienna Circle was concerned with guidelines for what is acceptable and not acceptable for a word (and concept) in science. Although this work has now evolved toward examining many issues within the philosophy of science, two issues were important from the beginning. The first was the clarity of the concept. This is often characterized by what you can point to or measure in order to identify the concept. The second was utility. This involved whether the concept could be related to one or more other concepts that describe separate events.

Among the various landmarks that reflect the evolution of this search for guidelines for scientific language, a few may be cited. Bridgman (1927) used the concept of operationism in physics and asserted that concepts should involve the description of operations that are used to measure them. S. S. Stevens (1935a; 1935b) and J. R. Kantor (1938) applied the concept of operational definition to psychology. The notion of operational criteria became applied to psychiatric nomenclature in 1980 (APA, 1980) with the *Diagnostic and Statistical Manual of Mental Disorders, Third Edition* (DSM-III). Much discussion continues about what components of definition and meaning should extend beyond the operations by which a concept is identified, but few have argued that the denotation of measurement has deterred the progress of science.

Guidelines have also evolved regarding diagnostic constructs (e.g., Cromwell, Strauss, & Blashfield, 1975). Diagnostic constructs are regarded as specialized types of scientific constructs. Accordingly, the criteria of clarity and utility are usually considered paramount. Four domains of data may be identified as possible contributors to the definition of diagnostic constructs: (A) historic/etiologic events, (B) presently observable events, (C) intervention (or prevention), and (D) prognosis (or outcome). Within these domains, the clarity of definition of a diagnosis would be determined by A and/or B. Utility would be determined by the extent that A and/or B predicts D, either with or without C. So, if schizophrenia (or any other diagnosis) is to be considered a useful construct, it should be clearly defined either in terms of (A) historic/etiologic events, and/or (B) currently assessable events; and it must be useful in predicting (D) outcome (on an individual or public health basis) both with and without (C) a specified intervention (i.e., a treatment or a preventive measure).

These guidelines afford a framework by which to view any diagnostic construct as it evolves. For example, only a very limited number of diagnostic constructs involve all four domains of data., i.e., A, B, C, and D. Only a limited number are defined in terms of data from both the A and B domains. At any given point in history, many diagnostic constructs involve no known treatment or prevention. In other words, they involve AD, BD, or ABD without the C domain. Few, especially those currently under investigation, have their ABCD relationships arranged in a linear or limited cause model; instead, the ABCD relationships must be understood in terms of a broader systems approach wherein the action of a given variable, be it A, B, C, or D, must be considered within the context of other variables also present.

These guidelines present a basis for evaluating the construct of schizophrenia and for discussing the chapter by Strömgren and comments made by McGlashan.[1] As a preface to their work it seems appropriate to say that schizophrenia, as currently defined in DSM-IIIR (1987), does not meet the guidelines just stated. The developers of DSM-III chose to focus upon operational criteria and their reliability; in particular, when two or more clinical judges viewing the same videotape (or other sample of behavior) from one interview occasion. Advances were achieved in this particular form of reliability for schizophrenia and other constructs, but little was accomplished for other aspects of reliability or for denoting utility (validity). This choice of strategy to develop and refine diagnosis is an unfortunate one, I feel, because it potentially freezes into place minimally reliable constructs with little or no validity. Progress would appear possible only when utility and clarity are advanced together.

---

[1]Dr. McGlashan's comments during the conference were based on a previously published paper (McGlashan, 1989). The reader is referred to this paper for the contents of his remarks.

Turning now to the preceding chapter by Strömgren and comments by McGlashan, a number of things are mentioned by them which may be analyzed in terms of the foregoing propositions. Comment will be focused here upon (1) the identification and relationship of basic to secondary features of schizophrenia, (2) the role of cognitive factors in the diagnosis of schizophrenia, (3) the role of reaction types or subtypes in schizophrenia, (4) the failing credibility of psychodynamic explanations of schizophrenia, (5) the specification of environmental factors, and (6) the role of omnipotence and positive self-attribution in normal and schizophrenic development.

What is Basic? What is Accessory?

A most salient issue comes from Professor Strömgren's review of Bleuler's development of the schizophrenia concept and his distinction between basic and accessory features. Even as a medical student, Eugen Bleuler had the advantage of being able to conduct many conversations with mental patients. German psychiatrists, "imported" to the Zürich area hospital when Bleuler was young, did not know the local dialect. Someone was needed to listen and understand more fully the comments and requests of the patients and to minister to their personal needs. Bleuler, as a medical student, was chosen for this task. This experience undoubtedly influenced him to describe and view schizophrenia from a subjective reference point more than anyone had ever been done before. Very likely also, he was influenced by the times. Philosophy, art, and literature were moving from a strictly rationalistic view of man to a more existential view which focused upon internal thoughts, feelings, motives, and conflicts. Political thought, meanwhile, was focusing more upon what is in the interest of the general welfare of all, including the common individual. Thus, Bleuler, more than anyone before him, came to describe schizophrenia in terms of the subjectively based referents of thought (internally held associations among words), affect (its coherence and its relation to cognitively experienced events), ambivalence (the decisionless tentative attribution of significance to things), and autism (the holding of private meanings or significance). It is within this context of subjective reference points, and inferences therefrom, that Bleuler viewed the basic features of schizophrenia. Accordingly, the externally based features of hallucination, delusion, and catatonia were viewed as accessory. Professor Strömgren mentions the implication by many that these are secondary to the "primary" basic features.

The basic vs. accessory distinction accompanied the coining of the word schizophrenia itself. Yet, the adoption and application of this distinction is yet to be resolved. Bleuler's 1911 treatise was not translated into English until 1950. While widely accepted as the classic work on the disorder of schizophrenia, it was essentially ignored by the makers of the DSM-III classification series. That is, the initial operational criteria in DSM-III emphasized the accessory symptoms (hallucinations, delusions, certain aspects of thought disorder) to define schizophrenia, quite the opposite of the symptoms Bleuler held to be basic. Moreover, symptoms that were primarily positive rather than negative were emphasized (e.g., see Cromwell, 1984). Both of these choices (of accessory and of positive symptoms) may have occurred because of the press toward identifying what would be maximally reliable (B domain) rather than what would be maximally relevant to prognosis (D domain) and to clinical decision and intervention (C domain). For whatever reason, however, the classification of schizophrenia in terms of "basic" features and the empirical antecedent-consequent relationships among defining features are yet to be fully researched. The construct of schizophrenia has suffered accordingly.

One may ask whether the results of the recent high risk (vulnerability) studies tell us anything about these basic versus accessory relationships attributed by Bleuler. If the high risk studies contribute anything at all, they suggest that attentional and information processing deficits (AIP+) may be primary, as a whole, to basic (primary), accessory (secondary), positive and negative symptom features of schizophrenia. In other words, the AIP+ signs are evident before the strictly clinical features of schizophrenia become manifest (Cromwell, 1984).

The prior assertion is based upon the research strategy that holds that much is to be learned from the mentally healthy relatives (offspring, siblings, parents) who have no sign of "unwanted" or schizophrenic behavior. A number of studies have now shown that these healthy relatives of the diagnosed patients have AIP+ features to an extent greater than that of either control subjects in the general population or control subjects who have been screened for absence of any family or personal history of psychopathology. Moreover, it has been shown in at least one study that it is the children with these deficits (as opposed to offspring of schizophrenic patients without the AIP deficits) who tend to break down as adults (Cornblatt & Erlenmeyer-Kimling, 1983).

What does this mean for the "meaning of schizophrenia?" It is difficult to argue that schizophrenia is a conjured illusion when predictions can be made about individuals who are genetically related but who show no defining signs of schizophrenia. However, it is also difficult to recognize definitions from a clinical interview, whether these definitions originate from Bleuler or from DSM-III-R, as being the ultimately useful ways in which schizophrenia should be described and defined. Instead, it may be that non-interview techniques assessing subtle aspects of cognitive and affective function must eventually play an equal role with interview in the delineation of what we call schizophrenia.

Turning to Dr. McGlashan's comments, I feel a similar issue emerges from his presentation of Sullivan's view of schizophrenia. In his interpersonal theory Sullivan sees psychopathology as originating with intolerable (not-me) anxiety at an early age, which leads, together with the adolescent surge of sexuality, to a "fracturing of the wall of selective inattention." According to Sullivan, when this happens self-integration itself fails, developmentally primitive states emerge, and an unpleasant sense of "nothingness" prevails. As may be suggested by the high-risk research cited above, the antecedent-consequent relationship of events may be misarranged in Sullivan's view. It may well be that the "fracturing" of attention occurs first, either because of genetic or unfavorable environmental factors that govern how the brain processes information. Following this may come the experience of trauma and anxiety, as the individual tries to process complex interpersonal information without the necessary resources. Only then, by mechanisms yet to be clearly identified, does the organism develop the manifest clinical features with which we currently define schizophrenia.

In describing Freud's two alternative views of schizophrenia, Dr. McGlashan not only presents a clear picture of a dilemma that Freud left unresolved (the alternative defensive and deficit views of schizophrenia), but he also reminds us how closely Freud's deficit view parallels the current view of how schizophrenia unfolds. He helps us understand how combined family therapy and pharmacotherapy are more effective than either used alone. The scenario that McGlashan recounts from Freud consists of (1) a withdrawal of libidinal attachments, then (2) a period of somatic and hypochondriacal preoccupation along with aggrandizement, then (3) a break in reality relationships, and finally (4) a projection of the internal collapse. This sequence of events is often, but not invariably, observed. It provides a dynamic basis for what is considered the treatment of choice today for most cases of schizophrenia: combined family therapy and pharmacotherapy. What Freud described as withdrawal is now typically described as the early negative symptoms of schizophrenia. Rather than being recognized as signs of mental illness, family and associates tend to view these as expressions of laziness (lack of motivation) and obstinacy. Thus, they are met with anger, frustration, and intolerance by the family and others. Then come the prodromal features, such as somatic preoccupation, which are likewise often misinterpreted by lay and, sometimes, professional parents. Next come the positive symptoms (the collapse), and now, usually for the first time, the family and friends recognize and accept that they are dealing with a mentally ill relative. Guilt, blame, and denial mix with the prior attitudes. The family pathology, in reacting to the mentally disordered family member, can be as distinctive as the mental disorder itself. Controlled research (Goldstein & Doane, 1985) confirm that combined family and neuroleptic drug therapy yields significantly better results than either one alone or than individual psychotherapy with neuroleptic therapy.

More recently, results have suggested that neuroleptic medication may relieve only the positive, not the negative, symptoms of schizophrenia (Spohn, Coyne, Larson, Mittleman, Spray, & Hayes, 1986). This finding confronts clinical researchers with the need for a new formulation of schizophrenia which can account for an aspect or kind of schizophrenia which is separate from the neuroleptically treated dopamine system.

The Role of Cognitive Factors

Professor Strömgren concludes that cognitive factors are of doubtful utility for diagnosis. Indeed, this may be the case. Most instances of cognitive deficit also occur with other disorders and are not specific to schizophrenia. Yet, in the same sense, delusions are not useful either; they also occur in a number of other disorders.

The major argument for cognitive deficit (referred to above more specifically as attention and information processing deficit [AIP+]) is that its various forms might lend an important insight to the genetic contribution to schizophrenia. A total of 45% of the normal healthy first-degree relatives of schizophrenics are reported to have smooth pursuit eye tracking deficit when asked to track a moving pendulum target (Holzman, Proctor, Levy, Yasillo, Meltzer, & Hurt, 1974). A total of 17% of the first-degree relatives of schizophrenics show reaction time crossover (DeAmicis & Cromwell, 1979). Such findings of failures in cognitive functioning may eventually be useful in identifying the phenotypes which clarify the genetic contribution to schizophrenia.

Reaction Types or Subtypes

Another unresolved issue which hangs as a cloud over schizophrenia research is whether it represents a single entity or is a group of relatively independent disorders with many common features during the final chronic stage. Professor Strömgren has referred to the paranoid vs. nonparanoid classification; the process-reactive classification is also commonly used. Sometimes the purported subtypes of schizophrenia can be explained away as being merely degrees of severity or different stages in the developing chronicity in a unitary disorder. Therefore, one crucial demonstration to justify subtype status has been for pre-identified subgroups of schizophrenics to fall in opposite directions from the normal control group. A number of such demonstrations have occurred: size estimation (e.g., Davis, Cromwell, & Held, 1967; Neale & Cromwell, 1968), incidental recall (Cromwell, 1968; Kar, 1967), numerosity (Schwartz-Place & Gilmore, 1980), and latent inhibition (Hemsley, 1987). However, the establishment of subtypes of schizophrenia on this basis remains elusive. One cannot distinguish between separate disorders and a single disorder afflicting individuals differing in cognitive style. Such cognitive styles may not be related to the disorder itself, but they may modify the way the disorder is manifested. Ultimately, the identification of distinct subtypes of schizophrenia may come when the ABCD guidelines, discussed earlier, are applied. In other words, multiple forms of schizophrenia would be recognized when separate identifying criteria (in terms of either historic or presently assessable events) lead to the usefulness of different interventions in order to gain favorable outcome.

The Failing Credibility of Psychodynamic Explanations

Strömgren and McGlashan both imply a role for psychodynamic, or at least psychogenic, contributions to schizophrenia. Professor McGlashan is forceful in his arguments as to why the psychodynamic view had lost credibility. Evidence of early parent-infant development or early trauma does not appear to occur in many cases of schizophrenia. Certainly, they do not appear to occur more often than in those patients with other diagnoses. Nothing can be formulated that accounts for the time lag between alleged early trauma and the adult onset of schizophrenia. Thus, the cure of schizophrenics through solely psychodynamic approaches is usually questioned. While the above statements are valid, a few Socratic questions may be offered to challenge whether the psychodynamic view should be discarded altogether.

Why is it that family therapy is so effective as an adjunct to neuroleptic therapy? One view is that the family therapy sessions provide the family a revised and more adaptive view of the mentally ill relative, and they are instructed in procedures of interaction and support that provide new attitudes and expectations toward the patient. One possibility is that the family therapy "takes the heat off" the patient, who has been coping not only with the illness but also with the hostility, criticism, rejection, and over-involvement of family members and friends. Indeed, the patient's behavior has been disappointing and unwanted. Another possibility is that social skills are being learned that allow the patient to cope with the family members. A third possibility is that changes are occurring in conceptual structure. Is it possible that the patient comes to construe the family and self in ways that are more adaptive than previously? Is it possible that superordinate constructs of understanding family members and people in general allow a level of conceptual integrity which had never before been achieved? If so, one could conclude that psychodynamics indeed play a role in the course and treatment of schizophrenia. Unfortunately, most current researchers of family therapy focus upon the family interactive features (expressed emotion, communicative deviance, affective style) rather than upon tracking the changes in conceptual structure in the schizophrenic patient as these therapeutic family events are taking place.

Why is it that the content of thought is not random during thought disorder? Clinical observation would suggest that sexual, aggressive and other emotionally laden content is associated more frequently with thought disorder than would be expected by chance. If this observation is correct, then Sullivan was right in his observation, though not necessarily in his interpretation. Primary process thinking of the parataxic and prototaxic sort emerges more often with schizophrenic thinking than one would expect by chance. In spite of the evidence for genetic contributions suggesting that cognitive AIP+ deficits provide a genetic vulnerability for schizophrenia, the cognitive errors that do occur often are fleeting fragments of sexual and aggressive thoughts that are normally warded off from attention. Until these selective thought disruptions are explained on another basis, it would seem unwise to discard a psychodynamic contribution to schizophrenia altogether.

The Specification of the Environmental Role

Strömgren's chapter and McGlashan's comments also bear upon the role of environment. Here, as well as in the genetics of schizophrenia, many issues are unresolved. A most convincing method to pinpoint the environmental contribution to schizophrenia is to identify differences which occur in monozygotic twins who are discordant for schizophrenia. All such differences would be environmental. For example, Reveley (1990) has found the affected twin to be lower in birth weight. Another method is to examine exogenous physical factors. In this regard, the hypothesis of prenatal viral insult has gained attention.

Most psychogenic environmental factors have focused upon stress. In fact, the stress-diathesis model is often taken for granted. It implies that stress is the crucial environmental contribution to schizophrenia. Perhaps it is time to question this assumption. Professor Strömgren, who cites the uniformity of incidence of schizophrenia throughout the world (regardless of endemic stressful conditions), apparently shares this view. As an alternative hypothesis, it is possible that uncertainty in conceptual structure (i.e., personal construct system) is the factor more appropriate than stress to join with the constitutional diathesis. Uncertainty would imply the lack of conceptual resources by which one could predict the outcome of one's own personal destiny in life situations. One might argue that this notion is not much different from that which is usually referred to as "stressful." However, uncertainty is a particular kind of stress. It implies that one has difficulty in predicting the outcome of positive, as well as negative, life events. If such a formulation of schizophrenia is useful, it would place added emphasis upon the research and understanding of cognitive structure. This possibility was suggested earlier when discussing family therapy.

The Role of Omnipotence and Positive Self-Attribution

The description by Dr. McGlashan of the model from Winnicott (a member of the British object relations school) is of particular interest in the current discussion, because it implies that the child, during the course of normal development, is indeed developing a personal construct system. McGlashan proceeds to interpret the Winnicott model as one that portends schizophrenia when events out of phase with the child's needs and states of activation bring about a premature destruction of the illusion of omnipotence. Increasingly, the needed omnipotence is derived from defensive, internal, or autistic fantasies rather than from external reality.

Although McGlashan describes Winnicott's model as one of the plausible, but now rejected, psychodynamic views of schizophrenia, it is also of interest because of its relevance to recent views of mood disorder. Mood disorder has been a diagnosis most difficult to distinguish from schizophrenia. In recent years, researchers have identified two important features that are specific to mood disorders rather than to schizophrenia. First, depressed individuals fail to show a 62% rate of positive evaluation of others, the "golden ratio" revealed by normal individuals regardless of language, age, and other factors (Dingemans, Space, & Cromwell, 1983; Space, Dingemans, & Cromwell, 1983). Second, normal individuals tend to view themselves more positively than the way in which others view them (Lewinsohn, Mischel, Chaplin, & Barton, 1980). If one uses the average view of others as the measure of objective reality, then the positive view of the self, observed in normal adults, is illusory. Since many of these positive evaluations involve power and control, normals can be assumed to have inflated "omnipotence." Depressives lose this omnipotent view. In short, the model presented by Winnicott may be more relevant to depression and other mood disorders than it is to schizophrenia.

Conclusion

Schizophrenia is a word. Like all words, the arbitrariness and change of definition has been evident. By the recognized standards for scientific and diagnostic constructs, the present definition of schizophrenia has clear limitations. This results partly from the absence of adequate data to determine the crucial events in the antecedent-consequent course of the disorder. It also results from the failure of the authors of recent nosologies to comply with utility guidelines, i.e., to select definitional features that optimize intervention decisions and prediction of outcome. This failure, however, does not justify a return to the pre-Kraepelinian era, in which very few individual difference constructs were useful in sorting out types of unwanted behavior.

Much of what has been researched in the psychology of schizophrenia has been generalized deficit, which occurs subsequent to the onset of the disorder. Since generalized deficit is a diffuse and general cognitive deficit, it does not justify the schizophrenia construct. To grasp the specificity of the schizophrenia construct, one must turn to two other areas of research involving schizophrenia. The first involves the documented instances in which schizophrenics or certain subgroups are, because of their disorder, superior in performance to normal individuals. (In addition to examples already mentioned, semantic priming is the most recent research example [Kwapil, Hegley, Chapman, & Chapman, 1990; Maher, 1983].) The second area, as already mentioned, is in the study of normal and healthy relatives of schizophrenics. Not only do they fail to show the socially "unwanted" behavior of the patient, but various reports have been made in which their behavior is superior to that of normal control subjects (see DeAmicis, Wagstaff, & Cromwell, 1986). In both cases, aspects of schizophrenia have predictive utility along dimensions that have nothing to do with unwanted behavior.

It is within the context of these issues that the meaning of schizophrenia is approached in Strömgren's chapter and McGlashan's comments. Each has approached schizophrenia with a view toward improving it by shedding some of our past misconceptions of the concept.

References

American Psychiatric Association. (1980). *Diagnostic and statistical manual of mental disorders, third edition*. Washington, DC: Author.

Bergmann, G. & Spence, K.W. (1941). Operationism and theory in psychology. *Psychological Review, 48*, 1-14.

Bridgman, P.W. (1927). *The logic of modern physics*. NY: Macmillan.

Cornblatt, B. & Erlemeyer-Kimling, L. (1983). Early attentional predictors of adolescent behavioral disturbances in children at risk for schizophrenia. In N. Watt, J. Anthony, L.C. Wynne, & J. Rolff (Eds.), *Children at risk for schizophrenia: A longitudinal perspective*. NY: Cambridge University Press.

Cromwell, R.L. (1984). Preemptive thinking and schizophrenia research. In W.D. Spaulding & J.K. Cole (Eds.), *Theories of psychosis: Nebraska symposium on motivation*. Lincoln, NE: University of Nebraska Press.

Cromwell, R.L., Strauss, J.S., & Blashfield, R.K. (1975). Criteria for classification systems. In N. Hobbs (Ed.), *Issues in the classification of children* (Vol. 1). San Francisco: Jossey-Bass.

Davis, D.W., Cromwell, R.L., & Held, J.M. (1967). Size estimation in emotionally disturbed children and schizophrenic adults. *Journal of Abnormal Psychology, 72*, 395-401.

DeAmicis, L. & Cromwell, R.L. (1979). Reaction time crossover in process schizophrenia patients, their relatives, and control subjects. *Journal of Nervous and Mental Disease, 167*, 593-600.

DeAmicis, L.A., Wagstaff, D.A., & Cromwell, R.L. (1986). Reaction time crossover as a marker of schizophrenia and of higher functioning. *Journal of Nervous and Mental Disease, 174*, 177-180.

Dingemans, P., Space, L.G., & Cromwell, R.L. (1983). How general is the inconsistency in schizophrenic behavior? In J. Adams-Webber & J. Mancuso (Eds.), *Applications of personal construct theory*. Ontario: Academic Press.

Goldstein, M.J. & Doane, J.A. (1985). Interventions with families and the course of schizophrenia. In M. Alpert (Ed.), *Controversies in schizophrenia*. NY: Guilford.

Hemsley, D.R. (1987). An experimental psychological model for schizophrenia. In H. Hafner, W.F. Gattaz, & W. Janzarik (Eds.), *Search for the causes of schizophrenia*. Heidelberg: Springer-Verlag.

Holzman, P.S., Proctor, L.R., Levy, D.L., Yasillo, N.J., Meltzer, H.Y., & Hurt, S.W. (1974). Eye tracking dysfunctions in schizophrenic patients and their relatives. *Archives of General Psychiatry, 31*, 143-151.

Kantor, J.R. (1938). The operational principle in the physical and psychological sciences. *Psychological Record, 2*, 3-32.

Kar, B.C. (1967). *Muller-Lyer illusion in schizophrenics as a function of field distraction and exposure time*. Master's thesis, George Peabody College, Nashville, TN.

Kwapil, T.R., Hegley, D.C., Chapman, L.J., & Chapman, J.P. (1990). Facilitation of word recognition by semantic priming in schizophrenia. *Journal of Abnormal Psychology, 99*, 215-221.

Lewinsohn, P.M., Mischel, W., Chaplin, W. & Barton, R. (1980). Social competence and depression: The role of illusory self-perceptions. *Journal of Abnormal Psychology, 89*, 203-212.

Maher, B.A. (1983). A tentative theory of schizophrenic utterance. In B.A. Maher & W.B. Maher (Eds.), *Progress in experimental personality research*, volume 12, (pp. 1-52). NY: Academic Press.

McGlashan, T.H. (1989). Schizophrenia: Psychodynamic theories. In Kaplan & Sadock (Eds.), *Comprehensive textbook of psychiatry*, 5th edition. Baltimore: Williams & Wilkins.

Mead, G.H. (1934). *Mind, self, and society: From the standpoint of a social behaviorist*. Chicago: University of Chicago Press.

Neale, J.M. & Cromwell, R.L. (1968). Size estimation of schizophrenics as a function of stimulus presentation time. *Journal of Abnormal Psychology, 73*, 44-48.

Reveley, A. (1990). *Twin studies at Maudsley Hospital*. Paper presented at the 1990 meetings of the American Psychopathological Association, NY.

Schwartz-Place, E.J. & Gilmore, G.C. (1980). Perceptual organization in schizophrenia. *Journal of Abnormal Psychology, 89*, 409-418.

Space, L., Dingemans, P., & Cromwell, R.L. (1983). Self-construing and alienation in depressives. In J. Adams-Webber & J. Mancuso (Eds.), *Applications of personal construct theory*. Toronto: Academic Press.

Spohn, H.E., Coyne, L., Larson, J., Mittleman, F., Spray, J., & Hayes, K. (1986). Episodic and residual thought pathology in chronic schizophrenics: Effect of neuroleptics. *Schizophrenia Bulletin, 12*, 394-407.

Stevens, S.S. (1935a). The operational bases of psychology. *American Journal of Psychology, 47*, 323-330.

Stevens, S.S. (1935b). The operational definitions of psychological concepts. *Psychological Review, 42*, 512-527.

5
Schizophrenia: A Medical View of a Medical Concept
Robert E. Kendell

Historical Background

The term schizophrenia was coined by the Swiss psychiatrist Eugen Bleuler in the early years or the 20th century. (Although his monograph *Dementia Praecox of the Group of Schizophrenias* was not published until 1911, the manuscript was completed in 1908.) As every schoolboy knows, the term means "split mind." It refers to the dissociation, or loss of coordination, between different psychological functions. Bleuler regarded this as the fundamental abnormality underlying the strange subjective experiences and behavioral abnormalities of the disorder. But although the term was Bleuler's, the original concept of an irreversible disease process with its onset in adolescence was Kraepelin's, and can be traced back to the 4th edition of his Lehrbuch (1893), published shortly after he moved to Heidelberg from Dorpat. In that 4th edition he described a group of what he called "psychic degeneration processes" (*Die Psychischen Entartungs Process*) which included Kahlbaum's *Katatonie* and Hecker's *Hebephrenie* and were characterized by the rapid development of a permanent state of "psychological weakness." In the 5th edition (1986) the name was changed to dementia praecox, a term originally coined by the Frenchman, Morel. Three major pathological forms, (hebephrenic, catatonic and paranoid), were described. At that stage in his career, Kraepelin regarded dementia praecox as a disease process which invariably resulted in permanent damage to the personality, in contrast to the disorders subsumed under his other great rubric, manic depressive insanity, whose individual episodes always resolved completely.

Schizophrenia, like its predecessors the psychic degeneration processes and dementia praecox, is therefore a concept: an explanatory and unifying concept that evolved in the imagination of two outstanding clinicians in an attempt to make sense of the shifting and variegated manifestations of insanity. Therefore, it can only be judged by the same criteria as other explanatory concepts—like natural selection, entropy, or migraine. It is meaningless to assert either that it does or that it does not exist. The only meaningful question is whether or not it is, or was, a useful concept—whether it succeeded in illuminating the shifting and variegated manifestations of insanity more effectively than other alternative concepts—and even this question has to be posed within a defined context. (Incidentally, Szasz' famous jibe that "schizophrenia does not exist" would have been equally meaningless had it been made in regard to tuberculosis or malaria. The organisms *Mycobacterium tuberculosis* and *Plasmodium falciparum* may reasonably be said to exist, but the diseases attributed to their propagation in the human body are concepts just like schizophrenia.)

At one level it is self-evident that schizophrenia is a useful concept, for the term has been used by psychiatrists throughout the world for three quarters of a century. On the other hand, its shortcomings are widely recognized. Its boundaries are not clearly defined, its etiology is largely unknown, and its validity is questioned by contemporary research workers like Angst (1988) and Crow (1987). Those to whom the term is applied are stigmatized both in their own and other people's eyes. There is therefore nothing inherently implausible in maintaining either that it does not delineate a valid grouping of patients and that some other way of classifying mental disorders would be preferable or, more fundamentally, that its parent concept of mental disease or disorder is inappropriate and misleading and that there are better ways of conceptualizing unusual subjective experiences and ways of behaving.

Diseases and Mental Disorders

Because schizophrenia is a concept of a "disease" or a "mental disorder," it must possess the characteristics of disease or mental disorder in general. Disease, however, is an imprecise concept, and mental disorder even more so. The term *disease* is not defined either in the World Health Organization's International Classification of Diseases or in textbooks of medicine. Dictionary definitions generally define disease in such terms as "an unhealthy condition" or "a disorder of body or mind." They are syntactical definitions providing rules of substitution rather than semantic definitions providing rules of application, and are therefore of little help.

Most physicians assume that when they or their colleagues identify a condition as a disease they are making an objective statement; they are irritated by people like King (1954) and Sedgwick (1982) who insist that they are simply making arbitrary value judgments. But if these same physicians are asked to explain why they regard some phenomena as diseases, and why they withhold this designation from others, it soon becomes apparent that they use different criteria on different occasions; at times they give the appearance of being prepared to employ whatever argument most conveniently provides the desired decision in each individual case. It is also clear that they have difficulty defining what they mean by "disease," dislike being asked to do so, and differ among themselves when they do succeed in defining the term. Such inconsistencies and contradictions raise the suspicion that "disease" is not a scientific term, or at least not one capable of exact definition. On the other hand, empirical studies of the phenomena labelled as diseases reveal a large measure of agreement, both among physicians themselves and between physicians and laymen. Almost everyone agrees that malaria, tuberculosis, lung cancer, and syphilis are diseases, and that drowning and starvation are not (Campbell, Scadding, & Roberts, 1979). (Incidentally, schizophrenia was rated as a disease in that Anglo-Canadian study by 92% of general medical practitioners, 78% of medical academics, 60% of non-medical academics, and 50% of secondary schoolchildren; higher percentages in each case than were obtained by hypertension or gall stones.)

In the 19th century mental diseases were widely assumed to be diseases of the mind, as opposed to diseases of the body, but the primitive Cartesian dualism underlying this distinction is irreconcilable with contemporary thinking in almost all the sciences concerned with cognition—psychology, neurophysiology, and artificial intelligence. Mental diseases are therefore to be regarded as a subset of disease in general, which do not differ in any fundamental respect from other diseases. Although it may still be appropriate in some contexts to draw a distinction between mind and body, and between mental and somatic events, it is important to appreciate that neither minds nor bodies are capable of becoming ill or "diseased" in isolation. Only people, or in a wider context, organisms, become ill or develop diseases; the most characteristic features of so-called bodily disease —pain and malaise—are subjective experiences. The only distinguishing features of mental diseases are their tendency to affect the subjects' cognitive processes, their perception of their environment, and their overall behavior; and the fact that the clinical manifestations of the disease are not easily referable to any individual organ. In practice, conditions tend to be classified as mental disorders if they are generally treated by psychiatrists. For example, in both the International Classification and the American Psychiatric Association's classification, Alzheimer's disease and anorexia nervosa are classified as mental disorders. But if the former were usually treated by neurologists it would be regarded as a neurological condition, and if the latter were usually treated by endocrinologists it would probably be regarded as an endocrine disorder.

The contemporary term "mental disorder" is virtually a synonym for mental disease. In the 1940's it was substituted for mental disease, partly in recognition of the increasing involvement of psychiatrists with a range of relatively mild departures from normality and partly in the hope that "disorder" —a term that is less explicitly medical —would be more acceptable to psychologists and other professional groups wary of medical hegemony. The American Psychiatric Association's current classification, DSM-III-R, comments that "no definition adequately specifies precise boundaries for the concept" of mental disorder, and then goes on to say that it "is conceptualized as a clinically significant behavioral or psychological syndrome or pattern ... associated with present distress or disability." It is also to be "considered a manifestation of a behavioral, psychological, or biological dysfunction in the person." Like the simpler dictionary definitions referred to above, this is essentially a syntactical definition providing rather cumbersome rules of substitution. It fails, perhaps deliberately, to provide a criterion for determining the status of controversial phenomena like alcoholism, homosexuality and persistent antisocial behavior. Although over 200 individual mental disorders are given semantic definitions providing unambiguous rules of application, mental disorder itself is not.

I have argued elsewhere that disease could, and perhaps should, be defined in terms of an objectively verifiable impairment of function, and that Scadding's "biological disadvantage" might serve as an appropriate criterion (Kendell 1975; 1986). Certainly, there is no doubt that many mental disorders, including schizophrenia, are associated with reduced fertility and reduced life expectancy and that either of these constitutes a "biological disadvantage." However, although I still believe that disease could be defined in this way, I am forced to concede that if one studies the way the term is used in practice, by doctors, it is difficult to avoid the conclusion that disease is not a biomedical concept at all, and that doctors do not want to have their freedom of choice restricted by a definition. Whether or not they admit or recognize the fact, "disease" is used by doctors themselves as a normative, or socio-political, concept. It implies simply that the condition in question is undesirable, and that on balance it is better dealt with by physicians and medical technology than by alternative institutions like the law (which would regard it as crime), or the church (which would regard it as sin) or sociology (which would regard it as deviant behavior).

Definitions of Schizophrenia

Kraepelin assumed, in the tradition of German academic psychiatry, that his dementia praecox was a disease entity, and that in time it would be found to have a specific aetiology and neuropathology, just as it had a specific symptomatology and temporal evolution. Bleuler made similar assumptions, except that his interests were in psychology rather than neuropathology and he assumed that the fundamental disturbance was a dissociation or loss of coordination between different "psychic engrams." Originally, therefore, the concept of dementia praecox/schizophrenia involved implicit assumptions about the aetiology of the syndrome. However, contemporary psychiatrists have been thoroughly persuaded by the arguments of Stengel (1959) and Hempel (1961) that if diagnostic terms like schizophrenia are ever to be used reliably they must be explicitly shorn of the kinds of etiological assumptions made by Kraepelin and Bleuler and provided with unambiguous operational or semantic definitions. For the last twenty years, therefore, schizophrenia has been defined by its clinical syndrome. In other words, that syndrome is schizophrenia.

The concept of a syndrome originated with Thomas Sydenham in the 17th century. It denotes a cluster of symptoms with a characteristic temporal evolution—to remit, to progress, or to recur. In the case of schizophrenia and most other mental disorders those symptoms are a mixture of abnormal or distressing subjective experiences (e.g., hearing voices) and observable abnormalities of behavior (e.g., blunting of affect). There is a broad measure of agreement on their identity and operational definitions like those of the Research Diagnostic Criteria (RDC) and Feighner criteria, and DSM-III and DSM-III-R, specify precisely which combinations of symptoms are adequate to substantiate the diagnosis. (Other subsidiary criteria like duration of illness, age, and marital status may also be involved, but symptoms provide the core of the definition in every case.) At least twenty operational definitions of schizophrenia have been published since the original Feighner criteria of 1972, and six or more of these remain in contemporary use. Although there is a core of typical patients who meet all definitions, there are significant differences in the populations of patients covered by each of these definitions, and each generates rather different values for the incidence of the disorder, its heritability, its responsiveness to therapeutic agents, and its prognosis (Stephens, et al., 1982).

None of these competing definitions can be said to be right or wrong, for as yet we have no external criterion of validity. If we were choosing between rival clinical definitions of Alzheimer's disease, we could pick the definition that most successfully identified those whose brains proved after death to have the characteristic neurofibrillary tangles and senile plaques found in that condition. If we were choosing between rival clinical definitions of Creuztfeldt-Jacob disease we could pick the definition that was most consistently associated with successful transmission of the encephalopathy in experimental animals. But where schizophrenia and most other psychiatric syndromes are concerned our understanding of their etiology is too incomplete for this to be possible. We can and should decide which definition accords best with traditional usage and which has the highest reliability. But we cannot decide which is most valid, for this would involve determining which of several different ways of defining the syndrome of schizophrenia most accurately picks out patients possessing the underlying abnormality we have not yet been able to identify. We therefore have to tolerate the simultaneous usage of several different definitions. This is, of course, rather confusing. But it is vastly preferable to agreement imposed by administrative fiat or political pressure; the coexistence of alternative definitions does at least serve to remind us that all definitions are arbitrary and liable to be changed in response to new evidence or arguments.

Schizophrenia is not alone in being defined by its clinical syndrome. The majority of mental disorders and many neurological disorders, like migraine and the dystonias, are also still defined in this way. Two hundred years ago most diseases were defined by their syndromes, but as knowledge about their etiology slowly accumulated they came, one by one, to be defined at some more fundamental level. The clinical syndrome "phthisis" became pulmonary tuberculosis, defined by the presence of tubercle bacilli in sputum or postmortem lung, after the discovery of the *Mycobacterium* by Koch; myxoedema became hypothyroidism, defined by the level of circulating thyroxine, when it became clear that the characteristic features of the syndrome were caused by a deficiency of thyroid hormone; and Down's syndrome became trisomy 21, defined by the presence of that additional chromosome, as soon as it was apparent that the syndrome was invariably associated with that chromosomal abnormality.

It is not by chance that most of the diseases that are still defined by their syndromes are either psychiatric or neurological. The human brain is a more complex mechanism, probably by several orders of magnitude, than any other organ of the body. It is hardly surprising, therefore, that we find it harder to unravel the etiology of its disorders and identify their pathology. There is no reason to doubt, however, that the etiology of schizophrenia will eventually be elucidated. Fundamentally, it is no different from any other disease. The evidence that genetic factors play a major role in its etiology is already beyond challenge (Gottesman & Shields, 1982) and evidence of a characteristic neuropathology affecting the medial structures of the temporal lobe is steadily accumulating (Bogerts, et al., 1985; Brown, et al., 1986; Crow, et al., 1989). Sooner or later, therefore, schizophrenia will come to be defined by its pathology rather than by its syndrome. Whether or not the name survives after this occurs remains to be seen, and is not a matter of any great importance. There are precedents both ways: "Gout" and "Down's syndrome" survived after their etiology was elucidated; "phthisis" and "Mediterranean anaemia" did not, though this does not mean that they were not useful and valid concepts in their day.

A more interesting subject for speculation is whether or not the boundaries of the new disorder defined by its pathology will correspond to those of the clinical syndrome we now recognize. It is frequently assumed that schizophrenia is etiologically heterogenous and that it will eventually be broken down into several subpopulations, some entirely genetic but transmitted by different genes, others largely or entirely environmental in origin, like the schizophrenic psychoses associated with temporal lobe epilepsy. By calling his monograph "Dementia Praecox or the Group of Schizophrenias" Bleuler clearly implied that this was his assumption; this has indeed been a common progression in medicine. Valvular disease of the heart, for example, was replaced by a range of different conditions like mitral stenosis and aortic incompetence, and Mediterranean anaemia was replaced by a bewildering variety of thalassaemias. It is also possible, though, that at least some parts of schizophrenia will be reunited with what we now regard as affective psychoses as a kind of reincarnation of Griesinger's *Einheitspsychose* (unitary psychosis). Schizophrenia and bipolar disorder share many characteristics and several contemporary research workers are beginning to wonder whether at least some of their determinants may be common to both (e.g., Crow, 1987).

The Boundaries of Schizophrenia

Kraepelin assumed that his "dementia praecox" or Bleuler's "schizophrenia" was a "disease entity." He did so, not because he had empirical evidence on that score but because from the middle of the 19th century until the middle of the 20th century most diseases were assumed to be entities with necessary causes that were either present or absent. This was because most of the great diseases that dominated medical practice in the 19th century—tuberculosis, syphilis, typhoid fever, cholera, and malaria—had been shown, one after the other, to be caused by infective organisms that were quite distinct from one another; it was therefore natural to assume that this was the nature of disease in general. Patients suffered either from tuberculosis or from syphilis, and although they might possibly have both infections simultaneously the causes of different illnesses were quite distinct. The mycobacterium did not shade into the spirochaete.

Unfortunately, most, if not all, psychiatric syndromes do shade into one another. In the first place, there are virtually no psychiatric symptoms which are pathognomonic of a single syndrome. The most characteristic symptoms of schizophrenia, Schneider's "symptoms of the first rank," are encountered in temporal lobe epilepsy and other brain diseases, and in amphetamine intoxication, and probably denote a relatively non specific malfunctioning of the deep structures of the dominant temporal lobe. Moreover, if two syndromes A and B are characterized by agreed constellations of symptoms a_1, a_2 ... a_r and b_1, b_2 ... b_r, it is always possible to find patients possessing a mixture of the two, e.g., a_1, b_2, b_3 ... a_r. The existence of interforms of this kind does not in itself invalidate the distinction between the two syndromes, any more than the existence of hermaphrodites and a variety of other well documented intersex states invalidates the distinction between male and female. It is crucial, though, that interforms should be relatively uncommon. The greys must not outnumber the blacks and the whites. There must be a 'point of rarity' between the two syndromes, which means in mathematical terms that the distribution of the scores obtained by a representative population of patients on a discriminant function, or some other linear function designed to discriminate between the two syndromes, should be bimodal. It must not be unimodal, with the scores of the majority of individuals lying in the middle of the distribution.

In the last thirty years many attempts have been made, either by discriminant function analysis or conceptually similar techniques like latent class analysis, to demonstrate "points of rarity" between one psychiatric syndrome and another. Some attempts have been concerned with mental illness as a whole, others with more restricted areas like the functional psychoses, affective disorders or depressive disorders. Regardless of the range of symptomatology investigated or the particular mathematical technique employed, most of these attempts have been unsuccessful. Either the original investigators were unable to demonstrate a bimodal distribution of scores or discrete clusters, or they failed to appreciate the need for cross-validation in a second data set, or other investigators were unable to replicate their claims. There is, however, one well designed study, based on ratings derived from a consecutive series of 500 patients and 1249 of their first degree relatives, which does demonstrate a convincing point of rarity between the syndrome of schizophrenia and other mental disorders (Cloninger, et al., 1985). Even so, there must still be some doubt whether the matter is settled, partly because the original symptom ratings may have been biased by the diagnostic preconceptions of the clinicians who made them, and partly because no other research group has yet repeated the demonstration.

The lack of discrete boundaries between different syndromes, or at least our inability to demonstrate their presence, is the source of many of our difficulties. This is why we are repeatedly driven to employing terms like schizo-affective disorder, mixed affective disorder, and borderline syndrome that embody an almost explicit recognition of interforms. This is also why the point at which psychiatrists have drawn the boundary between schizophrenia and the affective psychoses, or between schizophrenia and personality disorder, has swung backwards and forwards so alarmingly during the last fifty years. More generally, this is why we are unable to secure agreement on the definition of all our syndromes. If psychiatric symptomatology is continuously variable, and the statistical relationship between one symptom and another approximates a multivariate normal distribution, there is no good reason for placing boundaries in one place rather than another. Indeed, it would be more logical to abandon categorization altogether and use a dimensional classification instead. If, on the other hand, we could demonstrate points of rarity, or stable symptom clusters, the sites of those points of rarity and the boundaries of those clusters would themselves determine which combinations of symptoms were adequate to establish membership of individual syndromes like schizophrenia.

Relationship Between Syndromes and Etiology

Even if we ignore the paucity of the evidence that currently recognized syndromes like schizophrenia do correspond to natural clusters of symptoms with a characteristic prognosis, there is not in any case necessarily a one-to-one relationship between overt symptomatology and underlying etiology. Heart failure and anaemia are both well recognized and demarcated clinical syndromes, yet both are etiologically very diverse. Conversely, Huntington's chorea, which is known to be transmitted by a single dominant gene on chromosome 4, may be associated with a wide variety of psychiatric syndromes, including dysthymic, major depressive, schizophrenic and anxiety disorders (Caine & Shoulson, 1983). Whether or not the concept of schizophrenia corresponds to a natural cluster of symptoms and other characteristics, and is in that sense a valid concept, it does not follow that all schizophrenic illnesses share a common etiology. Indeed, the indications are that they do not. Even so, the history of medicine teaches us that an accurate identification of clinical syndromes greatly facilitates attempts to elucidate their etiology. Noguchi was only able to demonstrate that general paralysis was due to syphilitic infection of the brain because the alienists of the 19th century had been able to discriminate fairly accurately between general paralysis and other forms of insanity. Goldberger was only able to demonstrate that pellagra was due to a dietary deficiency because his predecessors had been able to distinguish pellagra from other psychoses.

The Present and the Future

The concept of schizophrenia retains its value for research workers trying to elucidate the etiology and pathogenesis of psychotic illness as well as for clinicians who need to be able to assess prognosis and to make rational choices between the different treatment strategies available to them. Few psychiatrists would be bold enough to predict that the term will still be in use in 50 years time, and it is important that research workers should continue to entertain alternative ways of classifying psychopathology. For most contemporary clinicians, however, the concept of schizophrenia remains invaluable and indispensable. It is woven into their ingrained ways of thinking; they would only be prepared to abandon the term if they acquired some dramatic new therapy that rendered old diagnostic distinctions irrelevant, or if the concept were undermined by radically new insights into the origins of psychotic illness. Despite the emerging insights of the last decade such developments are still probably some way off.

The Criticisms of Social Scientists

Although most thoughtful psychiatrists are well aware that schizophrenia is an imperfect concept that may well be discarded by their successors, they are, on the whole, singularly unimpressed by the criticisms of social scientists. To be told that schizophrenia is simply a form of deviant behavior is merely to be told what is blindingly obvious; it is no help to thought or action. Until social scientists are able to provide a convincing explanation of why the particular type of deviant behavior we call schizophrenia occurs throughout the world, regardless of major differences in language, religion, social structure and economic development (WHO, 1973), and with a remarkably similar incidence (Sartorius, et al., 1986), we will not take them seriously. Scheff and other labelling theorists have taught us something very important about the means by which people sometimes get trapped in careers as psychiatric patients, but they have not begun to explain the basic phenomena of insanity, schizophrenia.

We are not helped by being told that normal people may hold irrational beliefs or 'hear voices;' we know that perfectly well. Nor do we find it helpful to be told that we should listen to what our patients are trying to tell us rather than labelling them as hallucinated, deluded or thought disordered. We are well aware that patients' strange beliefs, and the peculiar subjective experiences they describe, are often comprehensible in the light of their cultural background and past experience. We will also admit that we sometimes place too little credence in what they say, or make too little effort to understand them. But it is vital not to confuse form and content. The content may indeed be meaningful and understandable. But it is even more significant that the idea is a delusion, and not merely an overvalued idea; that the hallucination is occurring in a setting in which other people do not experience false perceptions; and that the patient's difficulty in expressing himself coherently is not explicable in terms of limited vocabulary or education, or emotional arousal.

Too few of those who have contributed to the social science literature on schizophrenia have any extensive personal experience of the disorder. They are thoroughly familiar with the writings of other social scientists, and with parts of the psychiatric literature, but that is all. Psychiatrists have indeed said many silly things about mental disorders in the last hundred years, but at least their intimate personal contacts with their patients—the fact that they listen and talk to them and their families every week, and see at first hand how their lives progress from one decade to the next—puts limits on their absurdities. There are no such limits to the irrelevancies, absurdities, and plain misunderstandings generated by library-based theorists. Those who have the most intimate and extensive contact with the people psychiatrists label as schizophrenics—their parents, their brothers and sisters, their husbands and wives, and the nurses who care for them while they are in hospital—do not usually find the concept meaningless or unhelpful.

An effective critic needs to have some understanding of recent developments within psychiatry as well as some personal experience of the phenomena of mental illness if he is to criticize contemporary usage of terms like schizophrenia effectively. If he does not he is at risk of misunderstanding and misinterpreting things that are crucially important. Sarbin and Mancuso, for example, tried to validate, or invalidate, the concept of schizophrenia by reviewing "every article on schizophrenia published in the *Journal of Abnormal Psychology* for the 20 year period beginning in 1959" (Sarbin & Mancuso, 1980). Quite apart from the issue of whether it was sensible to try to validate a medical concept by studying the writings of another profession this whole enterprise was a waste of time, and well informed psychiatrists could have told them so in the 1970s. It is a sad historical fact that, under the influence of the psychoanalytic movement, the American concept of schizophrenia slowly expanded and degenerated in the 1940s and 1950s until it lost all sharpness of meaning and became simply a vague synonym for severe mental illness, casually applied to almost anyone who was ill enough to require admission to hospital or did not respond to psychotherapy. In the early 1970s the World Health Organization's *International Pilot Study of Schizophrenia* (WHO, 1973) and the US/UK Diagnostic Project (Cooper, et al., 1972) revealed how seriously American usage of the term differed from both its original meaning and contemporary usage in the rest of the world. (Russian usage was also idiosyncratic, though for rather different reasons). This led first to the introduction of the Feighner criteria by the St. Louis school (Feighner, et al., 1972) and eventually to the relatively narrow and precise definition of schizophrenia of the American Psychiatric Association's DSM-III (1980). The concept of schizophrenia on which most papers published in the *Journal of Abnormal Psychology* between 1959 and 1979 was based was indeed invalid. But this tells us nothing about the validity of contemporary concepts, or about the concept as it was understood in Europe and other parts of the world. Similarly, Dr. Coulter's observation that only about half the patients who met the imprecise DSM-II criteria for schizophrenia subsequently met DSM-III criteria is not evidence of the inherent shortcomings of the concept of schizophrenia. It is merely evidence of the magnitude of the adjustment needed by American psychiatrists and clinical psychologists in order to enable them to communicate with their colleagues in other countries.

The core of the concept of schizophrenia is the assumption that there is a biological difference, quantitative or qualitative, between those so labelled and other people, and that schizophrenics are fundamentally disadvantaged by that difference. The most important, though by no means only, element in the evidence for this biological difference is genetic; this genetic evidence is at the heart of the difference of opinion between psychiatrists and social scientists. Psychiatrists and geneticists are firmly convinced that they have demonstrated that genetic factors play a major role in the etiology of schizophrenia. The evidence of family studies in which relatives have been interviewed blind to proband diagnosis, of population based twin studies, and adoption studies all points in the same direction and is, in our judgment, incontrovertible (Gottesman & Shields, 1982). Anyone who tries to deny this evidence, whether they do so because they are unaware of the crucial studies, because they lack sufficient knowledge of human genetics to appreciate their significance, or because they are unwilling to accept that much human behavior is genetically determined, will simply be ignored by anyone with a biological training.

This is not to say that schizophrenia is a genetic disease like Huntington's chorea or cystic fibrosis, or that experiential and other environmental factors may not play a major role in its genesis. The fact that the concordance rate between monozygous twins is only 40-50% is evidence enough that they do. It is also apparent that what is transmitted genetically is a predisposition to develop a spectrum of disorders of which schizophrenia is only the most prominent, rather than schizophrenia per se. The mode of transmission and the genetic loci involved are also unknown. But the basic fact of genetic transmission is beyond doubt, and any social scientist who wishes to be taken seriously beyond the confines of his own discipline must come to terms with this fact.

References

Angst, J. (1988). European long-term follow up studies of schizophrenia. *Schizophrenia Bulletin, 14*, 501-513.

Bleuler, E. (1911). *Dementia praecox or the group of schizophrenias.* English translation by J. Zinkin, 1950. NY: International Universities Press.

Bogerts, B., Meertz, E., & Schonfeld-Bausch, R. (1985). Basal ganglia and limbic system pathology in schizophrenia. *Archives of General Psychiatry, 42*, 784-791.

Brown, R., Coulter, N., Corsellis, J., et al. (1986). Postmortem evidence of structural brain changes in schizophrenia. *Archives of General Psychiatry, 43*, 36-42.

Caine, E. & Shoulson, I. (1983). Psychiatric syndromes in Huntington's disease. *American Journal of Psychiatry, 140*, 728-733.

Campbell, E.J.M., Scadding, J.G., & Roberts, R. (1979). The concept of disease. *British Medical Journal, ii*, 757-762.

Cloninger, C., Martin, R., Guze, S., & Clayton, P. (1985). Diagnosis and prognosis in schizophrenia. *Archives of General Psychiatry, 42*, 15-25.

Cooper, J., Kendell, R., Gurland, B., Sharpe, L., Copeland, J., & Simon, R. (1972). *Psychiatric diagnosis in New York and London.* Maudsley Monograph No. 20, London: Oxford University Press.

Crow, T. (1987). Psychosis as a continuum and the virogene concept. In T. Crow (Ed.), *British Medical Bulletin, 43*, (Recurrent and chronic psychoses), 754-768. Edinburgh: Churchill Livingstone.

Crow, T., Ball, J., Bloom, S. et al. (1989). Schizophrenia as an anomaly of development of cerebral asymmetry. *Archives of General Psychiatry, 46*, 1145-1150.

Feighner, J., Robins, E., Guze, S., Woodruff, R., Winokur, G., & Munoz, R. (1972). Diagnostic criteria for use in psychiatric research. *Archives of General Psychiatry*, *26*, 57-63.

Gottesman, I. & Shields, J. (1982). *Schizophrenia: The epigenetic puzzle*. Cambridge: Cambridge University Press.

Hempel, C. (1961). Introduction to problems of taxonomy. In J. Zubin (Ed.), *Field studies in the mental disorders*, 3-22. New York: Grune & Stratton.

Kendell, R. (1975). The concept of disease and its implications for psychiatry. *British Journal of Psychiatry*, *127*, 305-315.

Kendell, R. (1986). What are mental disorders? In A. Freedman, R. Brotman,, I. Silverman & D. Hutson (Eds.), *Psychiatric classification*, 23-45. New York: Human Sciences Press.

King, L. (1954). What is disease? *Philosophy of Science*, *21*, 193-203.

Sarbin, T. & Mancuso, J. (1980). *Schizophrenia: Medical diagnosis or moral verdict?* New York: Pergamon.

Sartorius, N., Jablensky, A., Korten, A., Ernberg, G., Anker, M., Cooper, J., & Day, R. (1986). Early manifestations and first contact incidence of schizophrenia in different cultures. *Psychological Medicine*, *16*, 909-928.

Sedgwick, P. (1982). *Psychopolitics*. New York: Harper & Row.

Stengel, E. (1959). Classification of mental disorders. *Bulletin of the World Health Organization*, *21*, 601-663.

Stephens, J., Astrup, C., Carpenter, W., Shaffer, J., & Goldberg, J. (1982). A comparison of nine systems to diagnose schizophrenia. *Psychiatry Research*, *6*, 127-143.

World Health Organization. (1973). *Report of the international pilot study of schizophrenia, 1*. Geneva: W.H.O.

6
Schizophrenia and the Disease Model
Paul R. McHugh

In this chapter, I seek to clarify what I mean by the terms disease and model, what would constitute their proper application to any condition, their pitfalls, and advantages before I consider why their application to schizophrenia remains contended and what would be necessary to confirm this approach.

The Disease Concept

"Disease" is a very loosely employed term in many circles today and for many reasons. The most obvious laxity has been its drift into an all inclusive concept for disorder because of its success in the hands of clinician scientists in the last few centuries. I shall not recount the full history of that since I have documented it in the book, *The Perspectives of Psychiatry* (McHugh & Slavney, 1986). Through the efforts of individuals like Syndenham, Morgagni, and Koch, a program emerged for differentiating disorders and appreciating their underlying pathology and etiology. This program has been one of the most characteristic features of reasoning in modern medicine, but not the only one.

As a result of its source, however, the term "disease" has become identified with doctoring. Indeed, some would say disease is the only clear demarcating sign of medical responsibility. Therefore, anyone who speaks of disease is often stated to be using the "medical model" with its connotation of guild-like professional imperialism. However, the concept of disease is much more specific than disorder. There are many disorders that are not diseases and disease is not restricted to describing medical responsibilities. Rather, disease is to be identified as an organizational concept, a construct used to make sense of some disorders, and has quite specific operational criteria that direct attention along a pathway of research to validate or invalidate application of the disease construct.

Thus, the disease model is not the medical model, although doctors do use it, as well as other models, in their practice. Disease is not synonymous with the socially sanctioned "sick role," although it can be one of the best tickets of admission to that role.

Rather, disease is a term whose invocation should provoke an established path of questions and answers directed towards a foundational concept on which the suitability of the term will rest. The implication of concept is that when disease is present, the cluster of features of a disorder that represent the manifestations of the specific disease will--with a complete understanding--turn out to rest upon some structural or functional abnormality of a body part. Thus, at some crucial level of organization of the body, patients with a given disease will all be seen to share a distinct anomaly. It will be provoked by several different agencies, but it will, ultimately, help to explain both these patients' qualitative distinction as sufferers of the disease from the broadly construed normal population in which they are sequestered, and their remarkable resemblance to each other in the characteristics marking them as sufferers of the condition.

The operative words in this description are "complete understanding." Prior to that achievement, the ascription of the term "disease" to explain manifestations of disorder is hypothetical, unvalidated, and challengeable. The approach to construct validation applies here with vigor. The disease construct implies a constellation of manifestations in signs and symptoms caused by an underlying bodily pathological mechanism and cause. The validation of the disease rests not upon the reliability with which signs and symptoms can be observed, nor upon the subtlety with which they can be distinguished, but ultimately upon the development of empirical methods that can be used to investigate the underlying anatomical and pathophysiological domains from which the implied consistency of those signs and symptoms is derived.

Some disorders of the body and mind have been easily confirmed as diseases. When this occurs, research moves away from the early achievements of defining the cluster of symptoms in order to discern features of the underlying disruption of the brain or body, and moves on to study both how the anomaly in the body is capable of provoking the symptoms, and the genesis of the injury or abnormality based on an understanding of all aspects of the body as a biological entity.

A prototypic example is Huntington's disease, defined from its characteristic neurological and psychological features by George Huntington in 1872 and from its neuropathology, the fundamental abnormality of the bodily part (an atrophy of the corpus striatum) by Jelgersma in 1908. The contemporary investigation of Huntington's disease is quite lively. One aspect of this research is the study of the character of the dementia and affective problems displayed by patients in an attempt to relate those features to basal ganglia dysfunction. Another is the search for the gene responsible for the condition, located at the tip of the short arm of the fourth chromosome. Still another set of studies generated by the disease concept are ongoing investigations of molecular biology, seeking the mechanism behind the degeneration of the caudate cells and the onset of symptoms in middle life, an approach that offers opportunities for treatment and prevention.

This work represents disease reasoning at its best. In addition, it is worth noting that studies can go beyond the strictly biological aspects of the disease once it is clearly identified. Thus, the manner in which Huntington's disease can disrupt the family unit, and from that disruption provoke other difficulties such as delinquency and demoralization, has been a recent focus of research.

Reasoning about disease can be distinguished from much other work that doctors perform. The identification and study of deviance in mental deficiency and personality disorders which consume most psychiatric efforts is not, strictly speaking, the study of disease. The study of life burdens and the discouragement they produce in many individuals, and for which counseling is needed, is also not to be viewed as disease reasoning. Rather, disease reasoning is an attempt to define a specific kind of life burden and to come to appreciate it from the top down as signs of embedded bodily injury, and from the bottom up as the emergence of disruption from some misalignment of the constituents that bodies represent and that ultimately derive from DNA.

By this reasoning, our understanding of schizophrenia most resembles our understanding of conditions such as dementia, cerebral palsy, and epilepsy. All of these diseases are identified at first by some common cluster of symptoms, but are eventually appreciated as heterogeneous at several levels of the disease construct. They are heterogeneous at the level of manifest symptoms, pathology, and etiology. If the disease model is appropriate, then, with increased understanding, our knowledge of each condition will result in an appreciation of some damage to an intrinsic mechanism of the human brain essential to the smooth and proper functioning of mental life.

Schizophrenia and the Disease Model

Why should we think in these terms about schizophrenia, one could ask? Well, why shouldn't we think in these terms is perhaps a prior question, it seems to me. After all, over the last centuries, reasoning by disease has been the single most successful method of approaching anomalies in our understanding of physical disorders. It has provided the best answer to superstitions about such disorders as epilepsy. It acknowledges the vast ignorance that we have about the human brain-mind entity. At the same time, it offers a place to begin and a model to dispel some of this ignorance. It suggests that some disorders are "experiments of nature;" that if we explored for an anomaly of some brain part we could illuminate the roles and integration of brain elements.

On the other hand, and contrary to this call of tradition, the most telling reason to reject disease reasoning and this brain-based search for a pathological change in schizophrenia is that it has been the sinkhole of reputations for close to a century. Again and again the belief that we have been shown the pathology of schizophrenia turned out on closer inspection to be the result of some artifact of the preparation of the brain or some expression of the institutionalized life of the patients under study. With proper controls, the claims for the discovery of the pathology of schizophrenia have evaporated. This fact should hold a cautious person back from the disease model.

The second and most compelling reason, perhaps, to be cautious here is built into the term "model" itself. So far, my discussion has been about disease and not about modeling. Models have the great advantage of capturing certain critical aspects of a condition in a mechanistic way, and then displaying how these aspects can work in a dynamic interaction within a more complex system. If, however, the fundamental element within the model is not validated, then both the commitment to what the model seems to explain and the ease with which the model can be modified in the face of challenge can make it an obstruction to progress.

Models can be so fascinating that they blind one to alternatives. They are also very dangerous, since, at the same time, they can be perpetually modified in the face of new data and thus sustain themselves in a kind of irrefutable way. Models like the Ptolemaic System survived by employing the ingenuity of supporters to blunt criticism and by producing more supporters based on the general comfort of spurious knowledge than by empirical demonstration. Models should always remain, and be understood to remain, tentative until their predictions have been proven or disproven. And if long stretches of time go by during which the essential proof remains elusive, then the rejection of the model itself is often the only solution to free investigators to start again.

Difficulties in Reasoning About Schizophrenia as a Disease

Schizophrenia presents difficulties at many levels when disease reasoning is applied to it. First, it is difficult at the level of symptoms. The easiest entree to most diseases is the realization that the clinical particulars that form our diagnosis and that we wish to explain can be seen to fit together; they are conjoined in some fashion. A disease like dementia, for example, whose characteristics can be easily displayed, has symptoms all of which reflect aspects of the same underlying fact: the psychological disorder is one of decaying cognition. Similarly, delirium is a disorder of consciousness and manic depression is a disorder of affective life; in these cases, every identified symptom is really only a form of trouble in either consciousness or affectivity.

The symptoms of schizophrenia do not conjoin in this fashion. Disjunction is its essence. Any one symptom is capable of replacing another in the descriptive term "schizophrenia;" in no collection of symptoms is there some easily grasped central mental problem from which the positive symptoms, hallucinations, delusions, and thought disorder, or the negative symptoms of apathy and autism, seem to flow. Schizophrenia is difficult to describe and define even as a clinical concept beyond stating that it is an expression of insanity.

Any of the symptoms of schizophrenia can be a subject of argument over interpretation. Should it be construed as a particular form and evidence of injury, or rather as some functional attempt by the patient to make sense of a world of great distress to him? One cannot resolve this controversy by means of the mental symptoms alone. The term "symptom" itself seems to beg that question.

One is left with the hope that a lesion in the brain will either be discerned or excluded. It seems that only if disease is validated by such discernment can we come to appreciate the linkages within the variety of symptoms, and the distinctions between those symptoms, that are pathognomic of the disorder and those that are pathoplastic to the individual and his situation.

Again I shall argue by analogy. Pressing on with the disease model, I turn to its use and its initial difficulties in explaining epilepsy. It is clear that without an identified disorder in structure or function, the disease construct was unconfirmed in this disorder and was frequently challenged. This, however, did not make the ascription of disease irrational, mythic, or barren. In fact, as the example of epilepsy makes clear, the disease concept helped to stimulate discovery.

Epilepsy is now fully accepted as a disease, but it was questioned for many years because a whole variety of quite different appearing features were evident, and no pathology could be demonstrated in the brain of many epileptics. However, the mark of the 19th century in studying epilepsy was the recognition, first, that the most characteristic symptom could be construed as a sudden, repetitive stereotyped and excessive neural event—the ictus—and second, that many patients with epilepsy did in fact have clear pathological lesions of the brain - traumatic, inflammatory, and neoplastic.

This latter observation led to the happy distinction of symptomatic epilepsy (epilepsy based on a recognized brain lesion) from idiopathic epilepsy—a distinction known to Griesinger in 1848 and employed by him in the discussion of insanity. All these distinctions in epilepsy were eventually confirmed with the discovery of the EEG and the recognition that similar electrical discharges could emerge from a brain with crude injury (symptomatic epilepsy) or from one with no pathology discernible by the techniques we have on hand to characterize brain structure (idiopathic). A regular functional anomaly of the brain was evident in both groups from results of the EEG; this functional anomaly validated the application of the disease concept. The distinctive three per second spike wave complex of petit mal epilepsy gave clear assurance of a qualitatively distinct anomaly of the brain, confirming it as a disease.

Schizophrenia offers similar opportunities. There are many diseases of the brain that provoke clusters of symptoms that are schizophrenic-like. The classical ones are temporal lobe epilepsy and chronic pharmacologic doses of amphetamine and cocaine. Many others exist; the classic paper of Davison and Bagley (1969) gives a long list of different neuropathic conditions from which schizophrenic symptoms may emerge.

A recent observation from the NIH (Suddath, et al., 1990) that monozygotic twins discordant for schizophrenia show a diffuse ventricular enlargement in the affected twin suggests that a very subtle injury may lie at the root of many instances of schizophrenia. In my department, Barta, Pearlson, and colleagues (1990) have identified an atrophy of the left superior temporal gyrus and related that to the schizophrenic symptom of hallucinations.

Recently, in several different places, new forms of dynamic brain imaging have provided techniques for seeking anomalies of the brain that would confirm the concept of disease for schizophrenia. It was at Johns Hopkins that the suggestion of an excess of dopamine receptors as a fundamental aspect of schizophrenia was first proposed, based on the relationship of effective doses of phenothiazines to their dopamine affinity. This idea prompted a search with the PET scan of dopamine receptor density in schizophrenic patients. Larry Tune (Wong, et al., 1986) has gathered evidence for increased dopamine receptors. He admits that this is challenged by PET studies from Sweden with a different ligand wherein no increase in receptors was found. More investigation is needed.

Finally, etiology is crucial to disease reasoning. The search here goes on despite being stymied by the lack of a clear set of symptoms and a clear pathology. The genetic techniques of family studies, adoptive studies, and twin studies are all suggestive, but lack the regular requirements for a happy outcome: Mendelizing characteristics and identity in identical twins. The explanations for these failures are many. The need for life stresses to bring out what can be construed as an underlying vulnerability, as represented by the multi-hit concept or the diathesis-stress concept, has much to recommend it. However, many of these approaches worry all of us; they appear to be instances of playing with the model—adding the epicycles that make it work, rather than acknowledging that the model demands some intrinsic lesion representing at least one "hit" and carried in the word "diathesis." This needs demonstration rather than continual positing.

Schizophrenia is a mysterious condition and is likely to remain so for awhile. However, reasoning in terms of disease is lively today, particularly because new techniques for studying the brain have become available. In my opinion they are likely to be successful, ultimately, in confirming that there is a specific brain disorder that is necessary but not sufficient to produce schizophrenic symptoms. When that happens, the knowledge we will gain will extend beyond grasping what is specific and what is general in schizophrenia to a comprehension of some of the vital neural elements that lie behind normal and abnormal human mental life—the usual outcome of a successful analysis of the experiment of nature that diseases represent.

References

Barta, P.E., Pearlson, G.D., Powers, R.E., Richards, S.S., & Tune, L.E. (1990). Auditory hallucinations and smaller superior temporal gyral volume in schizophrenia. *American Journal of Psychiatry, 147*(11), 1457-1462.

Davison, K. & Bagley, C.R. (1969). Schizophrenia-like psychoses associated with organic disorders of the central nervous system: A review of the literature. In R.N. Herrington (Ed.), *Current problems in neuropsychiatry* (British Journal of Psychiatry Special Publication No. 4). Ashford, Kent: Royal Medico-Psychological Association, pp. 113-184.

Folstein, S.E. (1989). *Huntington's disease.* Baltimore: Johns Hopkins University Press.

Huntington, G. (1872). On chorea. *Advances in Neurology, 1,* 33-35.

Jelgersma, G. (1908). Neve pathologische befunde bei paralysis agitans und bei chronischer chorea. *Neurol. Zbl, 27,* 995-998.

McHugh, P.R. & Slavney, P.R. (1986). *The perspectives of psychiatry*. Baltimore: Johns Hopkins University Press.

Suddath, R.L., Christison, G.W., Torrey, E.F., Casanova, M.F. & Weinberger, D.R. (1990). Anatomical abnormalities in the brains of monozygotic twins discordant for schizophrenia. *The New England Journal of Medicine, 322*(12), 789-794.

Wong, D.F., Wagner, H.N., Tune, L.E., Dannals, R.F., Pearlson, G.D., Links, J.M., Tamminga, C.A., Broussolle, E.P., Ravert, H.T., Wilson, A.A., Toung, J.K.T., Malat, J., Williams, J.A., O'Tuama, L.A., Snyder, S.H., Kuhar, M.H., & Gjedde, A. (1986). Positron emission tomography reveals elevated D_2 dopamine receptors in drug-naive schizophrenics. *Science, 234*(4783), 1558-1563.

7
The Meaning of Schizophrenia: Compared to What?
John S. Strauss[1]

Compared To What?

A sociologist friend has had to remind me repeatedly that few things can be understood without considering their context. Piaget emphasized the same message, focusing especially on longitudinal context, the context of developmental trajectory. Although we tend to think of schizophrenia in its pure form with hallucinations, delusions, formal thought disorder, and perhaps abnormal affect, that is our abstraction. Schizophrenia never exists in a pure form. The focus of this chapter is that the person context is not trivial but is essential to understanding the meaning and nature of schizophrenia.

Bleuler provided many beautiful descriptions of the manifestations of schizophrenia. For example, he cited one patient who manifested a disturbance of association:

> Here in this smith-house it doesn't go very well. This is indeed no parish house or even a poorhouse, but in this place there is noise, anger, grumbling-sunny-heavenly-knells all year round. Many a small and large landowner, windbag or poor drunk from Thalweil, Addisweil, from Albis, from Salz, from Seen, from Rorbach, from Rorbas have never again returned to their own homes, etc., etc., etc. Greetings to all who are still alive. My own relatives no longer exist (Bleuler, 1950).

[1]The author wishes to express gratitude to Drs. Barbara Hanson, Larry Davidson, and to the persons with severe mental disorders who have participated in our research. This chapter is supported in part by NIMH grants #MH00340 and MH34365, a grant from the National Alliance for Research in Schizophrenia and Depression, and a grant from the Scottish Rite Foundation.

But as Bleuler also noted repeatedly, all the thinking of persons with schizophrenia is not so disconnected. For example, a patient with whom I worked had a diagnosis of paranoid schizophrenia and was often floridly delusional, sometimes manifesting formal thought disorder as well. Nevertheless, even shortly after demonstrating such symptoms, he could sit down and beat me at a game of chess. Another example of the range of behavior possible in a person with schizophrenia occurred during a large meeting that included professionals and people with schizophrenia and other severe mental disorders. One participant was seen pacing back and forth, looking disheveled, apparently talking to his voices, while others were engaged in the business of the day, such as planning programs. It seemed to me that this young man was very out of place in such a setting, being unable to interact reasonably with other people. As the meeting drew to a close, the planned entertainment began. It included a group of four musicians who played popular music. Shortly after they began, the young man who had been pacing and talking to his voices, went up to the bandstand, took over the microphone, and led the group effectively in an Elvis Presley song, singing the lyrics ("You ain't nothin' but a houn' dog") and indicating to each musician when it was his or her turn to play a solo. He was extremely skilled in this leadership role.

Even in those rare instances when it seems that the person is "nothing but schizophrenia;" if improvement occurs, he or she can often remember and recount with great clarity what the experience was like and what was happening in the surroundings. This phenomena has long been recognized in people who have experienced catatonic states, but it can be seen in other situations as well. For example, a young woman, a subject in our longitudinal study who had severe formal thought disorder that made it almost impossible to converse with her, began improving after several years. During an interview I had with her at the time of this improvement, she remarked, "I can talk more clearly now, can't I?" I replied, "Yes." She then continued, telling me how difficult it was before. She could tell that she wasn't making sense and that people were confused, so she would just withdraw, since there was nothing else she could do.

Such observations, as common as they are, do not fit easily into most of our conceptualizations. They indicate, for example, that schizophrenia is very different from an illness like a broken leg. You cannot break a leg, take off the cast in order to play football, and then, after the game, put on the cast again and be an invalid. With schizophrenia, health and illness exist side by side or can replace one another, even if not always completely.

Often the illness becomes more manifest at times of interpersonal or performance demand, but not always. The patient beat me at chess, after all. And if he did not see that as much of a challenge (which it wasn't for him), then we need to think about the role of personal meaning in helping to govern the process of shifting from function to dysfunction.

Perhaps even interpersonal demand is not so crucial. Although it is often believed that people with schizophrenia cannot relate to other people, especially when they are floridly psychotic, this too is an oversimplification. One patient in our study who was severely delusional seemed to put his delusions aside when he saw a fellow patient in distress. At such times he would reach out to comfort that person.

Schizophrenia is not like a fractured leg; it is not so simple. Even emphasizing diagnostic heterogeneity within "the schizophrenias" may primarily tend to distract us from a far greater aspect of complexity, the shifting from moment to moment or day to day, from ill to normal person. How is it that a "broken brain" (Andreasen, 1984) can function unbroken?

Subjective Experiences of Schizophrenia Revisited

The tendency to de-emphasize the variations, shifts, and co-existence of the normal and the abnormal in a person with schizophrenia in order to focus on "broken brains" and other notions implying permanent and massive biological dysfunction is furthered by the methods used for study and analysis. In our understandable efforts to describe problematic functioning and develop systems for clinical measurement, we have followed the almost universal trend of looking at small parts of the person's behavior. And explaining these parts has generated ratings that were often reliable. Thus, we can rate different kinds of thought disorder, abnormal perceptual experiences, and abnormal ideational content.

But in this emphasis on analyzing the pieces rather than the context, we may have ignored a major part of the picture. A few years ago, a woman physician who had contracted lupus wrote a series of poems about her experiences. These poems were published in *Psychiatry* (Kahler, 1987, reprinted with permission). The first page of this poetry is reprinted below:

Lupus, You Are a Queer Disease

When I was trying to be a wife, a mom, a doc,
life seemed so much simpler.
I was proud of giving.
"Go forth in peace to love and serve the Lord,"
didn't leave me with a resounding,
"How?"
Ideal or not,
my life was what I wanted.
Now I must receive.
Will my husband keep cooking?
I am not the woman he married.

My body—now too limber, now unbending,
one time pained, another numb
choosing at a whim false cues
from world and skin and self—
cannot move strongly now in the old ways
through water and through wind
over woodland miles,
nor wield as once
accustomed tools of craft and trade.
I'm trapped indoors by cold, pain, sun,
kept by erratic tiredness
that settles me content.
Slowly I let go old pleasures.
I don't look like a woman who ran 10K,
carrying her unborn passenger.
Friends, even my mother,
pass without recognizing me,
without refreshing my sense of who I am.
I have seen my face in the mirror
and not known who was there.

Pain makes me forget my old can-do self.
I feel strange among other people.
How can another person understand my pain?

This poetry, which in subsequent pages becomes cumulatively even
more powerful, has a very different feel from a rating scale for the
subjective experiences of lupus: pain (yes/no), depression (yes/no),
rigidity (yes/no). Perhaps it is acceptable to diagnose lupus as a
disease by such symptoms, as well as its various signs, since it is a

disease whose major manifestation is in the skin, kidneys, joints, and connective tissue. We know it primarily from these manifestations. However, schizophrenia is a disorder known primarily from its effect on the mind. If we insist on knowing it primarily through rating scales that focus only on small pieces of mental dysfunction, can we really know it? If we avoid talking with patients—as we frequently do— about the normal aspects of their functioning, about their views of how their illnesses have affected their lives, then we will systematically exclude such data from our consideration. When one does ask a person with schizophrenia how the disorder has affected his or her life, a very clear response will often be obtained: an awareness of the limitations that schizophrenia has imposed, and a description of an increased sensitivity to the suffering of others and understanding of that suffering are often mentioned.

Such molar considerations make the picture of schizophrenia more confusing of course. But by de-emphasizing these issues and the context they represent, we may have been "scientific" like the scientist who wanted to do a controlled comparison study of moose and bears. He first got a sample of moose and a sample of bears. And then to make the two comparable, he cut the antlers off the moose. To study a mental disorder and understand its significance, besides analyzing its components, it is also essential to note the entire human experience of the person with the disorder: their experiences of disorder and of healing, of functioning as well as dysfunction; and not to "cut off the antlers."

Thus, in considering schizophrenia, beyond considering looseness of associations, delusions, and other symptoms and signs, it is also important to consider statements such as the following:

> I'm in here, I got a problem, an illness, I'm in a mental hospital, I'm schizophrenic, still, I'd like to go to school. I've read a lot, took a course in parapsychology. The course in witchcraft, metaphysics ... Had to stop, the voices were learning what I was learning, it was coming back to me in a disorder. I was taking a course in astrology and had to stop it, I was teaching the voices too much ... I know this sounds crazy. Past four years, I never stayed out of the hospital over a year; a couple months, then I was in there for a month, and it's usually about this time of year when it starts. September to January, or March. Depends on how long I can put up with different parts of my illness. I told my new therapist, here it is, this time of year again, I don't know what it is, it's hard to explain, a feeling or a place, it's hard to put it together.

What is schizophrenic about how he describes his plight (in contrast to the symptoms themselves), you may ask. Exactly. These statements were made by a young man with paranoid schizophrenia who is overcome repeatedly by delusions and auditory hallucinations whenever he attempts to return to college. They reflect poignantly and reasonably his struggle to deal with his symptoms at the same time that he was attempting to attain his educational and other life goals.

Several years ago, a friend said to me, "You're the kind of person who, if it's raining, says 'look at all the air in between the raindrops'." Unfortunately, I wasn't as creative as he (it had never occurred to me) but the example was a good one. It is not possible to understand the manifestation of raindrops—their shape, even their existence—unless on considers their atmospheric context. Similarly, I think it is impossible to understand the disordered aspects of schizophrenia, unless we can understand how they co-exist with normal and effective functioning. How is it that a person with schizophrenia can say, as a study subject recently did, "Oh, I'm not being psychotic now. What I tell you [about her very high IQ] is true." How is it possible to interview someone with schizophrenia who begins to lapse into a formal thought disorder or delusional thinking and, after the clinician says, "I'm sorry, but I don't think we have time for that right now, I really need to know what's been happening to you," the person snaps back and returns to an accurate narrative description?

Schizophrenia, in its context, is not pure abnormality. It is the coexistence of disorder and order, of abnormal and normal. Viewed from this contextual perspective, the manifestations of schizophrenia reflect the interplay of cognition, feeling, and perception, and the way this interplay shifts in situations of comfort, repose, trust, perceived danger, and terror. Furthermore, it appears that this interplay shapes the course of disorder and improvement. One person with schizophrenia (real DSM-III-R schizophrenia) clarified for me the range of possible processes: healing, scarring, wasting time, learning to live with problems, spiraling downward.

How might these interactions between healthy functioning and dysfunction take place? Previous reports (e.g., Strauss & Carpenter, 1977) have identified reasons for believing that functioning in persons with schizophrenia and other severe mental disorders can best be understood in terms of open-linked systems. These systems, including symptomatology, social relations functioning, and occupational functioning, have been shown by prognostic studies to have their own longitudinal continuities, but at the same time to influence each other as well. Thus, for example, the best predictor of future work functioning is past work functioning, but past work functioning has some ability to predict future symptom severity as well.

The processes by which these systems interact are suggested by recent studies of pathways to improvement in schizophrenia. The concrete existence of reciprocal interactions is implied, for example, in observations of patients recovering from delusions (Sachs, Carpenter, & Strauss, 1974). It is possible to describe the improvement process in which the weakening of delusions seems to permit the patient to engage in more challenging activities. Success in those activities reassures the person and may give confidence, perhaps further reducing the intensity of delusions. As one patient in our study told us (this was a woman who had limited education and essentially no psychotherapeutic treatment), "I feel better about myself now so I don't have to be so paranoid any more."

Is it possible then that functioning can generate healing and healing can generate functioning, and conversely; that poor functioning, such as failure, can make the person more symptomatic? Although such relationships may exist and reflect a general principle, as in so many other aspects of severe mental disorder, the world does not appear to be that simple. We have suggested elsewhere (Rakfeldt & Strauss, 1989) that sometimes the very act of decompensation may be followed by increased pressure for the person to take hold and reorganize himself or herself. Returning to the broken leg analogy, it is as though decompensation for some patients at some times is like the refracturing of a poorly healed leg; if the rehealing process is followed by proper care, it may contribute to a more healthy overall recovery.

The context within which these interactions between function and dysfunction take place can be viewed (in a useful but conceptually flawed manner) as consisting of interactions between the person, the illness, and the environment (Strauss, 1989). This conceptualization is flawed because viewing the illness as existing separate from the person is problematic. Nevertheless, there are numerous valuable examples in subjective reports of schizophrenia by patients describing person-illness-environment interactions. Many persons with schizophrenia who have improved have cited the crucial role of a caring person, of someone who had faith in them (Deane & Brooks, 1963; Sechehaye, 1951; Strauss, 1989;). People with schizophrenia have also cited the helpful roles of structure (Leete, 1987) and work. Such interactions can set off sequences of functioning, increasing hope, reduced isolation from others, positive contact with others, self-esteem, and sense of mastery. All of these seem to influence each other in complex ways and may well contribute to healing processes. Strangely, much less is known about processes of decompensation, although it appears likely that similar interactions occur, although in reverse.

Patient reports about the interactions of function and dysfunction and about the role of the illness, the environment, and the patients themselves in these interactions are valuable; they provide such a common set of themes across time and across societies that one ignores them at great risk (a risk that has usually been taken). A kind of reliability has been demonstrated by these often similar reports and their frequency suggested a validity. However, it remains to be demonstrated that cause-effect sequences are actually at work here. The fact that more has not been done to determine whether such cause-effect relationships exist, given the huge amount of patient report data available, may be a sign of the degree to which these notions do not fit into dominant conceptual models in the mental health professions.

There are alternative explanations for why data that have been around since at least the early eighteenth century have not been taken more seriously. The patient reports could represent post hoc constructions by persons attempting to make sense out of a sequence that they could not otherwise explain in the same way that superstitions have been used in the past. At least some of the reports could be seen as only explaining the processes by which people begin to take hold of their lives and to function socially after the illness has somehow been diminished by other sources. However, accepting these "it's only" explanations without first exploring the possibility that what so many patients say is true would be a relatively unscientific approach. We would be comforting ourselves by fitting everything into current conceptual models rather than pursuing other possibilities.

The Meaning of Schizophrenia

In conceptualizing schizophrenia, various authors have considered different characteristics to be primary. Bleuler considered looseness of associations to be one of the fundamental features. Kraepelin described diminution of the will as a primary component. Contemporary focus tends to emphasize processes such as delusions and hallucinations, processes that earlier authors considered secondary. But perhaps schizophrenia is not based on a pathognomonic characteristic but arises from a process of growing dysregulation, a destabilizing system (Melges & Freeman, 1975; Strauss, 1987) in which, due to any one of a variety of problems, a relatively minor deviation feeds into another, which then amplifies the first deviation. This process involves ebb and flow, function and dysfunction, occurring in the same person and could be reversed or amplified, although we have only the roughest sense of the rules of such reversal or amplification.

If schizophrenia is dysregulation or a range of dysregulations of a complex system, then its etiologies can come at many points, as can sources of healing. Psychological, biological, and social factors in various combinations and degrees may play roles. But to move such a view beyond mere speculation, we must begin to delineate what these systems involve (Davidson & Strauss, submitted for publication) and the way in which various components influence their evolution. Otherwise we will be doomed to continue looking for the pathognomonic feature, the basic transmitter, structural brain defect, or psychological experience; chasing from one hoped-for answer to the next without pursuing the possibility that the answer consists of a complex range of features acting within the context of the person.

Is This Really Necessary?

If a "penicillin" to cure schizophrenia is discovered, then the above considerations are either wrong, or at least excessively difficult and not very important. Several types of pneumococcus, laboriously studied, have been demonstrated, but their existence became of little importance once the specific bactericide penicillin was discovered. I hope the penicillin for schizophrenia will be found, and that I will be proven wrong. But my hypothesis is that such a penicillin cannot exist because we are dealing with complex interactive processes, with many component causes unfolding over time, none of which is either necessary or sufficient. Furthermore, it seems likely that these processes are at the very core of human mental functioning.

The meaning of schizophrenia: compared to what? The meaning of schizophrenia compared to the person's competent functioning and the linked interactions between competence and dysfunction; this context may be the framework essential for understanding the meaning of schizophrenia and the processes involved in disorder and healing.

References

Andreasen, N. (1984). *The broken brain.* New York: Harper and Row.

Bleuler, E. (1911/1951). *Dementia praecox or the group of schizophrenias.* New York: International Universities Press.

Davidson, L. & Strauss, J.S. (submitted for publication). *Beyond the biopsychosocial model.*

Deane, W. & Brooks, G.W. (1963). Chronic schizophrenics view recovery. *Journal of Existential Psychiatry, IV(14),* 121-130.

Kahler, P. (1987). A new livelihood: Six poems. *Psychiatry, 50(4)*, 377-380.

Leete, E. (1987). The treatment of schizophrenia: A patient's perspective. *Hospital and Community Psychiatry, 38(5)*4, 486-491.

Melges, F.T. & Freeman, A.M. (1975). Persecutory delusions: A cybernetic model. *American Journal of Psychiatry, 132(10)*, 1038-1044.

Rakfeldt, J. & Strauss, J.S. (1989). The low turning point: A control mechanism in the course of mental disorder. *Journal of Nervous and Mental Disease, 177(1)*, 32-37.

Sachs, M., Carpenter, W.T., Jr., & Strauss, J.S. (1974). Recovery from delusions: Three phases documented by patients' interpretation of research procedures. *Archives of General Psychiatry, 30(1)*, 117-120.

Sechehaye, M. (1951). *Autobiography of a schizophrenic girl.* (Grace Rubin-Rabson, trans.) New York: Grune & Stratton.

Strauss, J.S. & Carpenter, W.T., Jr. (1977). Prediction of outcome in schizophrenia: III. Five-year outcome and its predictors. *Archives of General Psychiatry, 34*, 159-163.

Strauss, J.S. (1987). Processes of healing and chronicity in schizophrenia. In H. Hafner, W.F. Gattaz, & W. Janzarik (Eds.), *Search for the causes of schizophrenia,* (pp. 75-87). Berlin and Heidelberg: Springer-Verlag.

Strauss, J.S. (1989). Subjective experiences of schizophrenia: Towards a new dynamic psychiatry—II. *Schizophrenia Bulletin, 15(2)*, 179-187.

8

Schizophrenia: An Interpersonal and Kleinian Viewpoint

Elliott Jaques

The comments that are contained in this chapter are based on some points raised in discussions during the conference, and on my own background in psychiatry, the treatment of combat psychosis, and psychoanalytic theory. I will attempt to forge some links between seemingly disparate ideas in the hope of offering some new directions for thinking about the problem of schizophrenia.

Medicine, Disease, Linking, and Normality

Part of our difficulty in talking about schizophrenia is contained in certain implications of characterizing the problem as a disease, and in attempting to account for it by the use of medical models. One such implication is the extent to which schizophrenia crosses the boundaries of our usual conception of disease (Miller & Flack, this volume); that is, we presume that disorders in human beings are caused by somatic processes that can be alleviated by physical interventions. Medical interventions require medical qualifications, and a good part of the ideological debate over who should treat schizophrenic patients hinges on whether or not one defines schizophrenia as a somatic problem. This issue of the boundary between somatic and psychological territories has, of course, also been central to the debate over who is qualified to conduct psychotherapy. As is well known, even though Freud (1926) felt that nonmedical professionals should be entrusted with the psychotherapeutic care of patients, our own American Psychoanalytic Society has balked at qualifying anyone without an M.D.

In any case, the history of the concept of schizophrenia is one in which the phenomenon has bounced back and forth between the medical and nonmedical sides of our clinical and theoretical fences.

More often than not, this has resulted in a splitting off of one ideological camp from another, each getting at certain aspects of the phenomenon while remaining adamantly blind to other aspects, with the result that few fully realize the complexity of the problem. Part of the difficulty, then, is the way in which we have gone about trying to solve the problem. If we are going to come to grips with the problem of schizophrenia, we are going to have to find meaningful ways to work both sides of the fence. This will entail dealing with enormously complex issues, such as those referred to by John Strauss (this volume) and others.

Before we can make a meaningful start on such a project, it would seem that we need to take one step backward to clarify a crucial point raised by a number of authors in this book. In our discussions of schizophrenia as a disorder, it has been recognized that the meaning of order, or normality, stands in need of clarification. On the medical side of the fence, the meaning of abnormality is assumed to entail dysfunctions in the organism that prevent effective social functioning, and that can be put right by physical intervention. This appears fairly clear until we come to consider behavioral disorders such as schizophrenia. I think that at least one of the reasons why schizophrenia is such a difficult problem to grasp is that we have great difficulty getting straight what we mean by social normality. Of course, this is not a problem peculiar to psychiatrists and psychologists, but one that wreaks conceptual havoc with sociologists, anthropologists, and other social scientists as well.

The issue of defining normality and, by implication, abnormality, is one that Daniel Miller and I have been working on for about 25 years. In order to get a feeling for what psychology might mean by a normal person, we have found ourselves asking what ethics means by an ethically sound person, what the religions mean by a moral person, and what law means by a reasonable person. Interestingly enough, in each case the answers lead us to the same type of person. That is, what seems to be common to each way of thinking about normality is the ability to interact effectively in social encounters, what Miller (Flack & Miller, 1991; Miller & Jaques, 1988) refers to as the capacity to fulfill the social prerequisites (Aberle, et al., 1950) of a society.

One aspect of this thinking that I want to draw attention to is that when we are talking about people in social situations, we are talking about their ability to link, to get to-gether, to resonate with each other. This is associated with linking intrapsychically (Bion, 1957), that is, with mental processes that are linked and integrated, and with the satisfying experience of interacting with others on the basis of trust.

I would like to underscore this point by a brief digression into etymology. In contrast to linking, when we talk about schizophrenia, we are talking about splitting (Bleuler, 1911/1950; Klein, 1946). Likewise, far from finding interaction, in schizophrenia we observe withdrawal. Similarly, in contrast to trust, in schizophrenia we find suspicion and paranoid thinking. All told, schizophrenic features of behavior are precisely the opposite of what we consider to be the characteristics of constructive social encounters.

Looking still further into the etymological roots of terms associated with a good society and good social interaction, consider ideas such as justice, freedom, and liberty. These constitute an interesting confluence of concepts. Etymologically, "trust" comes from "troth" and "tryst," related to "betrothal," and "marriage," themselves tied up with "truth," —all very closely linked constructs in human thinking. "Justice" comes out of the Latin "jus," joining together, (the base of the word "jury"), in contrast to "injury" and the splitting, disjoining, and disjunction that we are concerned with in schizophrenia. "Freedom" comes via a Germanic root from "abode," and the idea of the descended family living in trusting relationships in an abode, as opposed to the withdrawal that is so characteristic of schizophrenia. Finally, "liberty" is associated with love and loving relationships, in contrast to the anxiety about love, loving relationships, and destructiveness in schizophrenia. In sum, what we think of as normal has to do with the ability to take part in good, trusting human relationships, which is in total contrast to schizophrenic problems, which center on the inability to take part in trusting and close encounters with others.

In a nutshell, it seems that one way of arriving at a useful definition of schizophrenia, one means of demarcating its boundaries, is to start by considering universal characteristics of social behavior and social interaction. I suggest that when we are talking about schizophrenia, we are not talking about the reflection of some specific kind of entity or disorder, but rather about a reflection of universal and fundamental features of all human life that depends on encounters with others.

Vulnerability, Combat Psychosis, and Melanie Klein's View of the Paranoid-Schizoid Position

One explanation of schizophrenia that has enjoyed much popularity in recent years is the vulnerability hypothesis, usually associated with Joseph Zubin (Spring & Zubin, 1976; Zubin, Steinhauer, & Condray, this volume). Implicit in Zubin's model is the notion that we are all subject to the possibility of a schizophrenic breakdown. The basic idea seems to be that with either sufficiently high stress or degree of vulnerability, one traverses the line between sanity and psychosis. Some individuals (presumably those who are more vulnerable) go over the boundary with little stress, whereas others (presumably those are who are less vulnerable) go over only after experiencing the greatest degree of stress.

This is precisely what one saw in combat psychosis during the second world war. Individuals whose histories gave no indication of schizoid symptoms reacted to battle conditions by breaking down into what any of us would diagnose as a gross schizophrenic reaction, including delusions, hallucinations, and utter confusion. Within three days after coming out of combat, the psychosis lifted; there was complete remission and no recurrence of symptoms or residual effects.

The vulnerability model implies that this kind of breakdown could well occur in a large proportion of the population, given a comparable degree of stress. One implication that may be drawn from this argument is that we are talking about generalized developmental patterns and behavioral phenomena that can be included within the limits of the definition of schizophrenia given earlier. A second implication is that the etiological factors at work in schizophrenia are multifarious. Although there is certainly a constitutional or genetic underlay, it is apparent that there is no *single* necessary factor that is crucial.

This set of ideas can be related, I think, to theoretical developments in psychoanalysis, particularly object relations theory in Britain.[1] Influenced by the developmental theory of Melanie Klein (1975), one group of analysts in the U.K., including Wilfred Bion (1957), Herbert Rosenfeld (1987), and Hanna Segal (1981), has been engaged in understanding and treating schizophrenic patients. It seems to me that Klein's model of early infant development is closely related to some of the points discussed earlier.

Klein's (1946) theory of earliest infancy (the first 6 to 12 months of life), is concerned with the active participation of infant and mother in social interaction or, from the point of view ascribed by Klein to the infant, the breast-infant relationship. It is important to note that the situation is not merely one consisting of the mother or infant in

---

[1]Until very recently, many discussions of object relations theory have cited Fairbairn and Winnicott, while neglecting the seminal work of Melanie Klein (e.g., McGlashan's discussion during the Clark conference). Unfortunately, Klein's theory, and even mention of her name, have been anathema in psychoanalysis in this country for many years.

isolation, but one consisting of an interaction between the two of them. Klein posited that the development of a tendency toward schizophrenia begins as a predisposition in the infant toward experiencing very intense destructive impulses, on the one hand, and a mother who finds it difficult to cope with her infant's destructive behavior (such as attacking with the hands and mouth). A failure to resolve the interplay among associated factors such as love and hate, the good and bad self, and the good and bad mother, leads to splitting. Such splitting, a defensive maneuver against phantasied annihilation, is the basis of later schizoid processes in adulthood. In these, love and hate are split from each other, the world is made up of either good objects or bad objects, the good self or the bad self, and ambivalence and guilt are avoided in an effort to ward off the experience of depression. The point, for present purposes, is that this process is posited as part of the development of each one of us, and that we employ the residues of these early experiences as a means of coping with stressful situations. Klein (1975) maintains that maturation and normal development entail the satisfactory working-through of these early experiences, resulting in what she calls the depressive position, wherein the infant becomes capable of coping with ambivalence and tolerating anxiety and guilt (assuming that all goes well).

Again, this account is meant to provide a particular kind of model of ordinary development in all human beings. To a greater or lesser extent, each of us works through these early processes; subsequently, we carry within us the possibilities that—given enough stress—the unresolved aspects of these early conflicts, in which splitting and other schizoid mechanisms are used to alleviate anxiety, could be reactivated.

In conclusion, I would only add that there are a multiplicity of ways in which we cope with and unload many of these conflicts in ourselves. Much of what underlies some of the unattractive aspects of social life, such as prejudiced behavior, mistrust, and paranoia between social groups, can be accounted for by this way of thinking. In other words, rather than a discrete phenomenon such as that explained by a discontinuous theory of developmental stages, Klein's notion of positions implies that schizoid behaviors and ways of thinking operate along a continuum of vulnerabilities to which we are all subject.

To bring the argument full circle, the proposition is that in schizophrenia we are dealing with behavioral patterns common to, and potential in, all human beings. Each of us is capable of using schizoid mechanisms in our social relationships and, given sufficient amounts of stress, we are all capable of breaking down as well.

References

Aberle, D.F., Cohen, A.K., Davis, A.K., Levy, M.J., Jr., & Sutton, F.X. (1950). The functional prerequisites of a society. *Ethics, LX* (2), 100-111.

Bion, W.R. (1957). Attacks on linking. *International Journal of Psycho-Analysis, 40,* 308-315.

Bleuler, E. (1911/1950). *Dementia praecox or the group of schizophrenias.* NY: International Universities Press.

Flack, W.F., Jr. & Miller, D.R. (1991). Social interaction and schizophrenia: Problem, theory, and research. *Schizophrenia Research, 4*(3), 303.

Freud, S. (1926). The question of lay analysis. *The Standard Edition of the Complete Psychological Works of Sigmund Freud,* Vol. 20, p. 183-258.

Klein, M. (1946). Notes on some schizoid mechanisms. *International Journal of Psycho-Analysis, 27*(3), 99-110.

Klein, M. (1975). *Envy and gratitude and other works 1946-1963.* London: The Hogarth Press.

Miller, D.R. & Flack, W.F., Jr. (this volume). Defining schizophrenia: A critique of the mechanistic framework.

Miller, D.R. & Jaques, E. (1988). Identifying madness: An interaction frame of reference. In H.J. O'Gorman (Ed.), *Surveying social life: Essays in honor of Hubert H. Hyman.* Middletown, CT: Wesleyan University Press.

Rosenfeld, H. (1987). *Impasse and interpretation: Therapeutic and anti-therapeutic factors in the psychoanalytic treatment of psychotic, borderline, and neurotic patients.* London: Tavistock Publications.

Segal, H. (1981). *The work of Hanna Segal: A Kleinian approach to clinical practice.* Northvale, NJ: Jason Aronson.

Strauss, J.S. (this volume). *The meaning of schizophrenia: Compared to what?*

Zubin, J. & Spring, B. (1977). Vulnerability—a new view on schizophrenia. *Journal of Abnormal Psychology, 86,* 103-126.

Zubin, J., Steinhauer, S., & Condray, R. (this volume). *Schizophrenia From an American Perspective.*

9
The Trouble with Schizophrenia
Joseph Margolis

Strategies of Analysis

The general disarray in recent efforts to formulate a convergent and economical model of schizophrenia suited to the work of professional therapy and the findings of the principal medical, sociological, and allied disciplines ought not to be regarded as evidence of an incipient mass schizophrenia on the part of the members of the affected specialties. It is really nothing more than a sign of being entirely in touch with the prevailing high-level disputes in the philosophy of science (particularly in the philosophy of the human sciences) and with even larger disputes regarding the cognitive intransparency of nature and the horizonal bias of the history of cognitive inquiry. The full significance of this connection with other fields is very largely ignored. In fact, it is entirely predictable that well-informed specialists in schizophrenia, (chiefly psychiatrists and behavioral scientists), who tend to form distinctly opposed theoretical camps among themselves, would probably join forces to greet the supposed diagnostic relevance of such conceptual issues with a good deal more than genial doubt.[1] They would be mistaken in doing so, however. The quarrels in the field are not merely disputes about alleged findings regarding neurophysiological deviances or patterns of social formation; they concern the very logic of disease and mental disorder.

It is clear that we may be easily sidetracked by the enormous questions raised about the definition of schizophrenia, so that we do

---

[1]Surprising as this may seem, it is confirmed by the underlying "empirical methodology" common to such completely opposed conceptions of schizophrenia as are developed in McHugh and Sarbin, (both this volume). Taken together, these two chapters give a fair sense of the characteristically (or at least occasionally) extreme opposition between psychiatric and behavioral-science conceptions. On the argument being mounted, it is not a question of which is more nearly right as it is of the bearing of deciding which is right on the strength of a methodological finding about *how* to investigate the question.

indeed ultimately ignore the diagnostic issue (and a fortiori, the therapeutic issue); for example, by becoming absorbed in questions regarding the proper nature of medicine, the logic of medical and behavioral norms, the very idea of objectivity, the prospects of the physical, biological, or behavioral reduction of mental, social, and cultural life, the proper modeling of science, or the import of cultural and historical relativity.

No doubt these are important matters, and no doubt their resolution does bear in a substantive way on a final formulation of schizophrenia. But to yield too much or too quickly in their direction would be to fail to give due dialectical weight to other large conceptual considerations that are plainly crucial to the theory of schizophrenia, and particularly to the notion of what we should mean by the use of the term. You may take this as a piece of friendly philosophical diagnosis regarding our own quite agreeable form of professional disorder.

Having set these niceties aside, we may identify at once the source of the deepest uneasiness about all accounts of schizophrenia, namely, that there is no generally agreed-upon theory of persons or *selves*—to whom the schizophrenic condition is rightly ascribed, if ascribed at all; and that there is no promising schema for theorizing about the nature and structure of persons or selves that can be expected to yield in a direct way any fine-grained genetic, neurophysiological, physical, biochemical, behavioral, psychodynamic, informational, functional, or other mapping of the intrinsic processes of molar persons or selves (as such). The pertinence, and even the decisive importance, of all such somatically centered findings is certainly not being put into question by admitting the above point. The question, rather, is just *what* is the relevance of such findings? There simply is no reasonably stable conceptual picture of the self common to all the sciences that can be expected to anchor our debates about psychiatric or behavioral disorders (which are explicitly characterized as disorders of the normal integrity of the self's structure or of its normal mode of functioning). This is not quite true of such seemingly closely linked conceptual distinctions as those of depression (e.g., Wiener, 1989) and neurosis (though they surely have their own difficulties, which are bound to touch at some point on the deeper concerns that are being raised here); but for obvious reasons it *is* true of such categories as multiple personality and borderline personality disorders—that is, weak-boundaried ego-functions and weakly entrenched individuating ego-identity functions (Hamilton, 1988; Rinsely, 1982).

These reflections help to bring into conceptual relief the differences between three quite general strategies of analysis that may be applied to schizophrenia: treating schizophrenia as a disorder of, (1) functioning molar persons as such; (2) limited, quite particular affective, volitional, and doxastic functions distinctly more peripheral and less global than those of the first option; and (3) some definitely submolar or somatic functioning—possibly biochemical or neurophysiological—that characteristically manifests itself symptomatically at the level of molar functioning. It is entirely possible that all three strategies may be differentially productive in different sectors of therapeutic interest, and may even be integrated into a coherent and inclusive theory.

Now, it is a mistake to think that the weakness mentioned—in theorizing about the nature of science itself—is merely a sign of the primitive state of any particular science. It might be better viewed as a sign of the enormous conceptual power of those same sciences—not altogether unlike, perhaps, the significance of our failing to achieve a completely unified theory of all forms of physical force. For, all things considered, the form our theory of the self takes is, effectively, the form of our entire theory of man's relation to his encompassing world.

That may seem a bit of purple prose until we realize that it is quite impossible to characterize schizophrenia (as it is now generally viewed) in any terms weaker than those that address at least one's cognitive orientation within, and one's mode of processing information about, the entire order of intelligible reality. To admit that much is already to admit a very strong theoretical bias favoring strategy (1).

It takes very little reflection to appreciate that the legitimacy of the very enterprise of science is under no circumstances thought to be merely one technical or internal question among others, one that any particular scientific discipline could answer. Therefore, the modeling of the self is not (or not in all pertinent regards) merely a technical question for a specialized science. It is, rather, an undertaking that attempts to bring into comprehensive and unified order *all* of our best clues about the nature of cognitive endeavor, the sources of distortion or defeat of such endeavor, and the production of behavior said to be congruently informed by such inquiry. This, in short, is an analogue of the essential difficulty of theorizing about schizophrenia in terms of the first strategy.

Put another way: if we favor the first strategy, then schizophrenia must be one of a very special array of clinically significant disorders. It can no longer be regarded as a mere first-order medical or behavioral syndrome of any sort. It remains an empirical matter, all right. But it now appears to be a disorder that implicates our second-order (or critical or legitimative) reflections on our intrinsic cognitive competence. Perhaps the right analogies to invoke are relativity and quantum physics; the late developments in physics are also impossible to pursue in any merely first-order terms: the well-known paradoxes of relativizing simultaneity and of the indeterminacy of location and measurement at microtheoretical levels confirm that there is no conceptual disjunction between physics and the theory of knowledge. Correspondingly, the medicine or behavioral science that addresses schizophrenia thus characterized is conceptually and methodologically different from what it might be supposed to be if its paradigm cases were, say, more like Down's syndrome or depression, or bulimia.

We cannot expect our theory of intact, normal, integrated persons to be better than our theory of effective science, our theory of what is real in nature and human culture, or our theory of what counts as an appropriate adjustment in our forms of inquiry set to discern the actual structures of reality. If we select the first strategy, then a theory of schizophrenia is tantamount to a theory of science, knowledge, or intelligence. Nothing less will really do. Furthermore, since we are well aware of the perplexities of ever getting such a theory right, we must (according to the argument) concede the extremely tentative, even prejudiced, nature of our theory of selves or persons—*a fortiori*, our theory of schizophrenia. Put in just these terms then, *any* diagnosis of schizophrenia that construes it as a disorder of persons or selves and, therefore, as a disorder involving cognition and thought processes related to those processes that produce science itself, will *in some large measure* be a disorder of learned or socially acquired competences (however genetically, biochemically, or neuro-physiologically enabled). Therefore it will to some extent elude the disease (or "medical") model in which schizophrenia would be construed in somatic terms alone, or in terms that (however somatically affected by learning and thought processes) are not themselves thought to be disorders of the learned processes of cognition and thought. In short, by this argument—and it is a very modest argument—strategy (3) *cannot* afford an adequate or correct account of schizophrenia.

Our theories of science inevitably skew our notion of the normal functioning of the self, by virtue of which schizophrenia is viewed as a distinct disorder. Theorists are naturally disposed, therefore, to begin to build their account of the self and of schizophrenia in such a way that this tendency becomes an internal feature of the very model they mean to defend. Theories of normal and schizophrenic functioning tend, therefore—if we reflect on the horizonal, culturally relativized nature of our inquiry into cognitive competence—to be themselves cast in terms of culturally relativized normality. This, of course, affects the prospects of our second strategy for analyzing schizophrenia, and also depression and neurosis (e.g., Miller & Jaques, 1988; National Institute of Mental Health, 1987).

The point to bear in mind is that, although the adjustment is inescapable, it may take an equivocal form. For, according to the general argument being sketched, the disease model of schizophrenia also cannot escape being culturally relativized, even though it presumably eschews or marginalizes the cognitional dimension of the disorder; which is to say, its own presumptions of objective validity are culturally skewed in an insuperable way (given the conceptual connection between theorizing about schizophrenia and theorizing about the conditions of true knowledge). However, the model that construes schizophrenia in terms of normal social functioning (and not, or not merely, in terms of some submolar somatic functioning) builds that relativity into the very structure of schizophrenia itself. If you admit that much, then you have decisively altered the very nature and methodology of psychiatry—*if* psychiatry is supposed to be the discipline of choice in diagnosing and treating schizophrenia. The connection is ineluctable.

There is still a fundamental difference, of course, between models of these two sorts: for instance, one may emphasize biochemical imbalances and the other, deviant behavior. But those differences may also obscure any (further) effective convergence regarding social relativity and its bearing on our model of the self—on the condition of failing to grasp the deeper conceptual connection between theorizing about the self and theorizing about disorders of the self.[2] That is, if schizophrenia is a disorder *of the self*, and if selves are culturally emergent sites of cognitive and related competences, then the theory of schizophrenia will reflect the peculiarly reflexive bias with which we regard ourselves (within the terms of the variable horizons of different cultures, taken either synchronically and diachronically or both). Something of the sort will affect all science, to be sure. But the failure to reduce the concept of the self to the relatively lawlike regularities associated with purely physical phenomena signifies a conceptual difficulty that is essentially neglected: the avoidance (when one is theorizing about normal and abnormal psychological states) of the normative bias of our home society. (On the other hand, of course, if schizophrenia were not characterized as disease or disorder of the self, then, of course, some promising correction of such bias may well be forthcoming.)

If, as now seems reasonable in the light of the largest puzzles about knowledge, there *is* no reliable sense in which scientific objectivity is

---

[2]In a fair sense, *this* is the clue to the profound error in the provocative account offered a good many years ago by Szasz (1961). Cf Margolis (1966).

simply progressively approximative of the structures of reality—
particularly where the structures of human and cultural life are
concerned—then differences in the treatment of cultural relativity, as
between, say, medical (or, better, disease) and social-functional models
of schizophrenia, are bound to be somewhat illusory and misleading
(Margolis, 1986). To the extent that schizophrenia *is* a theory of the
functioning of molar selves—and that is still its principal focus,
though it is entirely possible (as we have already suggested) that the
term is no more than a blunderbuss for a variety of discrete, even
modular submolar syndromes—*there can be no avoidance of
relativized norms of functioning*. There are, of course, promising
studies that indicate distinctive metabolic patterns of frontal lobe
activity among schizophrenics. These patterns might well be
disengaged from theories that strongly depend on the functioning of
molar selves; that is, theories in which functional symptoms lead us
to theorize about relatively independent patterns of brain activity (e.g.,
Buchsbaum & Haler, 1987). In that case, theorizing about medically
distinct somatic patterns classified as, or as part of, a complex
syndrome still to be delineated as schizophrenia (or to be separated
from its ancestral form) may eventually enable us to deny any central
role to disputed theories of the self. They could all, in principle,
become otiose on both conceptual and empirical grounds. But we have
no promising conceptual option before us that could actually effect
such a change. Gains along genetic, hormonal, neurophysiological and
related lines are genuine enough; but their mere accumulation does not
affect the issue in the least. A conceptual revolution is needed.
Schizophrenia and its derivatives would then behave, conceptually, in
a way more comparable to depression and somatically defined
disorders than, say, to multiple personality. This possibility favors both
our second and third strategies. Nevertheless, saying that obliges us to
consider more closely just what may be said about modeling the self.
Here, we must face the fact that the line of demarcation between
medical, somatic, disease, and related theories of schizophrenia and
blatantly philosophical theories of the self begins to fade. There is a
seamless continuum between the one and the other that may be
ignored at our conceptual peril.

The point is a nagging, even an irritating, one. There are any
number of different strategies for theorizing about schizophrenia. They
are all affected, as is the whole of science, by theorizing about the
very conditions of what we are prepared to denominate as science.
That question is hardly a specialized question, a question for a
particular science. It is now known to be a peculiarly contingent
matter that directly and differentially affects the substantive work of
any particular science—especially if we concede (as is now

everywhere granted) that: (a) science cannot be separated from its own history; (b) nature is cognitively intransparent; and (c) our own mode of inquiry and the legitimation of our inquiry are comparatively blind artifacts of our own historical situation. Add to this the further fact that the theory of what we are to count as knowledge and as the intelligent use of knowledge is, at bottom, *also a theory of the human self*—or at least of that functionally integrative capacity (cognition) that is at the heart of our theory of the self. It cannot, then, fail to strike us that *all* our medical, psychodynamic, behavioral, and related theories of schizophrenia focused on the normative or normal function of molar selves are merely the inverse of the state of our present theories of cognitive competence, whatever else they may be. That much is ground zero for any molar theory of schizophrenia, and *a fortiori* any theory of affective, volitional, or characterological disorders, or of submolar somatic disorders of the relevant kind; that is, *of disorders that are in some essential way informed by learned or socially acquired cognition and formal thought processes.* The reasons are that schizophrenia is construed as a disorder of molar selves (in the fullest sense in which we theorize about the self) and that diagnostic medicine and its cognate therapeutic disciplines are addressed there (one way or another) to the largest integrative functioning of human persons. These themes are notoriously ignored or deprecated professionally. The question is not merely one of turf: it is rather a question of the elementary coherence of *any* pertinent diagnostic and therapeutic discipline.

The Self and Schizophrenia

Let us concede the point, then, and turn to its more detailed payoff for the theory of schizophrenia. What I now offer is a very brief list of the most serious conceptual findings and options regarding the theory of the self that are bound to bear in a most substantive way on our local theories of schizophrenia:

(1) the concept of the self is, indissolubly, the concept of the active site at which the symbiosis of cognized world and cognizing competence obtains;

(2) the concept of the self is not a natural-kind concept, since the concepts of truth and knowledge, themselves essential to defining the self, are not natural-kind concepts; that is, it is impossible to construe the self as functioning merely in accord with *any* set of the covering laws of nature—although saying that does not entail

that the self functions in a contracausal way or in a way that positively violates any admitted laws of nature; hence, it cannot be the subject of any straightforward science of the usually supposed canonical sort;

(3) the concept of the self's normal functioning is a speculative projection of how the somatic and behavioral possibilities of the species *Homo sapiens* can, within the cognitive constraints of a contingent science and a historically and culturally skewed general understanding, serve the perceived interests of given human societies (themselves historically constructed and not generable in any known way from any mere *natural-kind* considerations);

(4) the self is a culturally and historically formed (or constructed) cognitive and active site able to instantiate any of a wide range of behavioral and mental conditions favored by and congruent with the perceived interests of the society in which it is thus formed and from which it emerges. Hence, there is a natural congruity between such formed and formative processes; even the would-be correction of the self's molar functioning (when deviating from the norm) and the confirmation of the very concept of what it is to function as a normal self are artifacts of the inherent horizonal limits of a particular society's cognitive vision. Even scientific objectivity and the notion of natural norms are artifacts of that same condition.

These four items have quite radical implications that go to the heart of what we may understand as a scientific psychiatry or behavioral therapy and that have a bearing on the diagnosis and treatment of schizophrenia. But there is a further family of distinctions very closely related to the foregoing (but of even more substantive importance for the theory of schizophrenia) that bears out the warning offered earlier on, namely, that there is no reliable disjunction between high-level medical theories (as well as theories of allied sorts) and what must be frankly conceded to be philosophical speculations about the nature of the self. By "philosophical speculations," we mean a kind of theorizing that may be conceptually "fitted" to the salient empirical facts of any discipline but that cannot yield in any familiar way to straightforward empirical confirmation or discomfirmation, processes which are usually thought to obtain crisply in somatic medicine or other physical and biological sciences. What is decisive here (although often overlooked) is that this conceptual "addition" is not merely an enlargement of the context in which we appreciate the ramifications of psychiatric or behavioral-science intervention: it substantively and differentially affects the empirical work of such disciplines.

The four items offered so far are certainly stubbornly philosophical in this respect. I claim that these are essential considerations in attempting to define schizophrenia. But saying all this is *not* meant to deny the characteristic rigor of psychiatry, of diagnostic and therapeutic disciplines, or of philosophy itself. It is, on the contrary, meant only to disabuse us of certain naive or hopelessly sanguine views of what we might otherwise suppose a scientific medicine or therapy to be.

Let us add a few more items that capture the most troublesome features of any attempt at an objective theory of schizophrenia:

(5) the concept of selves or persons, unlike the concept of *Homo sapiens*, is the concept of a certain kind of historically or contingently variable cultural agent; hence, it is a concept of a family of such viably different agents, all compatible with the biological regularities and capacities of *Homo sapiens* but exhibiting distributively different, even opposed and irreconcilable, forms of functioning organized in accord with different norms, habits, technologies, institutions, practices, interests, and theories about the whole of man's cognitively—informed life;

(6) the concept of the self is the concept of a historically open-ended range of possible modes of functioning that cannot in principle be brought within the confines of any totalized schema of all viable possibilities governing the normal or normative relationship between *Homo sapiens* and historically evolved persons; the adjustment of the category of schizophrenia to that of normal functioning is and must be forever hostage to the evolving forms of historicized human life itself. In principle (in the relevant diagnostic and therapeutic sense) these forms can never be brought under the conceptual conditions of a relatively closed science; the very forms of human history are not generable from any known alphabetic conditions from which known historical societies may be thought to be generated.

All this is entailed by the seemingly modest claim that the self is not a natural-kind term. It confirms that the three alternative strategies for analyzing schizophrenia that we originally laid out do not yield merely alternative nosologies: they are, rather, profoundly different methodologies and ontologies. That is what is usually overlooked in the familiarly cantankerous disputes between psychiatrists and behavioral scientists. Theorists of these sorts are often disinclined to suppose that their empirical disputes are also second-order disputes. But they *are*.

We need not, let us be clear, slight, deny, or ignore *any* of the valuable findings of a diagnostic medicine that contributes to our understanding of the somatic conditions of schizophrenia: the only question we are raising concerns the conceptual relevance of such findings *to that diagnosis*. That cannot be settled by any first-order medicine or behavioral science. Furthermore, we need not deny that it remains entirely possible in principle to outflank *all* the foregoing argument by demonstrating the preferability of strategies (2) or (3) or, more fundamentally, by providing a satisfactory reduction of the concept of the self to somatic terms. Thus far, neither option is sufficiently compelling, and neither is conceptually obligatory.

It may help to say that items (5) and (6) are the most radical consequences derivable from a general reading of science or by way of reading something akin to Thomas Kuhn's (1970) *Structure of Scientific Revolutions* along the lines of Michel Foucault's (1977) radical conception of cultural history. But, in saying that, we emphatically do not want to suggest that these items, any more than the first four, depend in any essential way on the doubtful details of either Kuhn's or Foucault's theories. The references are meant only as a convenient means of orientation.

The final item that is needed in our list is possibly the most problematic.

(7) the concept of the self is the concept of a *functional* unity, not a *substantive* one, fitted to the functional norms of a particular society or fitted transculturally but still from that society's perspective; that is, it is the concept of a complex mode of functioning that can be localized (as belonging to a particular member of *Homo sapiens*) and that, as such, meets in some measure the requirements of the operative norms and interests of the society in which the self emerges—but without requiring (or being shown to require) any single substantively unitary node underlying such a functional unity.

In short, the self is not, and does not entail, a soul, an essential ego, a transcendental mind, an executive homunculus, or anything of the kind in order to ensure or explain the (functional) unity of all its processes. On the contrary, whatever may be empirically best suited to account for memory and forgetfulness, unconscious process, dissociation, hypnotic and paranormal conditions, habituation, modular functioning, distributed and hierarchical order, and every loosening of conventional notions of the self's substantive unity, are entirely compatible with what we are here calling functional unity. For example, a viable surviving multiple personality, amnesiac, or the like is unified enough for our present purpose.

This conceptual economy is welcome, of course, given the known empirical difficulty in locating the self introspectively, and given the need to avoid any of the conceptual scandals of a dualism of mind and body. But the price we pay is also severe. For, according to this argument, there cannot any longer be a substantive distinction (a distinction regarding the essential or lawlike properties of some determinate substance) between normal and schizophrenic functioning. There cannot be a detectable disorder in some material or immaterial substance (neurophysiological, say, or Cartesian) in terms of which to fix, for the first time, the disorder we call schizophrenia. If we restrict ourselves to our first strategy then schizophrenia can only be a functional disorder that accords with items (1) through (6) *one that cannot be radically different in principle from the mode of functioning we call normal*—at least as far as the notion of unified functioning is concerned. Modular somatic disorders can only be local, in our terms, *conceptually* subordinate to a culturally defined mode of functioning. In short, the argument entails that there is an irreducibly ideological dimension to our theory of schizophrenia.

There would still have to be what we may call the *unicity* (or numerical unity) of the self to consider. There would have to be some minimal *functional unity* of that numerically distinct self to acknowledge—effective, affective, conative, doxastic, or intentional. But there would not have to be, and according to the argument there could not be, any *substantive* (somatic—neurophysiological, say) *unity* of the self to explore, by virtue of which an objective distinction between normal and schizophrenic states of the self could be defined. If that now means that there cannot be an "objective" medicine or an "objective" cognate discipline concerned with disorders like schizophrenia, so be it. But the conclusion is unnecessarily severe and unrealistic. It would be much better to change our conceptions of what *is* objective than to ignore or discard the kind of rigor that is possible in these disciplines. So a review of the theoretical status of schizophrenia is, effectively, a review of the very status of science and medicine.

Levels, Constructions, Disjunctions and Distinctions

Three rather large findings may be drawn from the foregoing. First of all, the diagnostic concept of schizophrenia appears to entail second-order philosophical (or legitimative) concerns in a distinctive way: the disorder itself is conceived as centrally assigned to the cognitive powers of functioning selves, and knowledge is a peculiarly disputed notion that cannot be characterized in natural-kind or somatic terms. It is, on the contrary, peculiarly affected by the generally admitted intransparency of nature and the historically emergent and socially constructed nature of human selves. Second, a change in the concept of schizophrenia along the lines suggested directly entails a change in the concept of what it is to be a science and, more specifically, what it is to be a science addressed to the diagnosis and therapeutic treatment of schizophrenia. It would not, for example, be able to be reconciled with the familiar unity-of-science or inductivist models that have dominated the theory of science from the time of the Vienna Circle to very nearly the latest pronouncements in the Anglo-American philosophy of science centered in the work of, say, Carl Hempel (1965). And third, the functional unity of the self required and posited in any account of normal functioning apt for defining the disorder that is schizophrenia does not require that the self be more than a functionally identifiable site of such functioning, that its characteristic features not be assignable to socially learned processes of functioning, that those processes not be widely variable among historically viable societies, and that any somatic determinants of pertinently normal and deviant functioning not necessarily be conceptually subordinate to the use of a diagnostic category centered on socially learned functioning. Since, of course, *no* functioning of the sort in question can obtain without being incarnate in somatic processes, there cannot be any reasonable disjunction between a somatic medicine and a behavioral science bearing on schizophrenia; such a medicine or science can never be adequate if one is disjoined from the other.

Of course, all this is contingent on there being no satisfactory restriction of schizophrenia to the range of disorders that could be collected under our original second or third options. Perhaps it will be useful to add three further distinctions—implications, as it happens, of the foregoing account, but still too busy to permit elaboration here—that would have to be adequately explored if we were ever to convince ourselves we had arrived at a full understanding of schizophrenia.

The first concerns the "inter-level" nature of the theory of schizophrenia, apart from the first-level/second-level complication already remarked. That is, assuming a failure of reductionism, schizophrenia, like biological evolution, cannot be characterized in the terms of any reasonably satisfactory "same-level" empirical inquiry, regardless of the model of such an inquiry. If one takes physics or chemistry or molecular biology as models of a science that confines its descriptive and explanatory terms to one level of discourse (admitting that, in another sense, descriptive and explanatory discourse may also introduce a distinction of "levels"), then there is no prospect at present that medicine could be such a discipline. Hence, the peculiar complexity of the diagnosis of schizophrenia generates an additional problem for a discipline that is already characterized as moving between genetic or molecular processes and molar interaction between organism and environment (and this, of course, implies the existence of endlessly many functionally defined processes linking whatever is specified regarding molar organisms and molecular processes).

Another distinction of importance concerns the profoundly historicized, culturally emergent, or constructed nature of the self and its artifacts and distinctive forms of functioning. This consideration is bound, in principle, to baffle any pretense at universally invariant covering laws—though not, for that reason, the bare pertinence of causal factors. To the extent that the notion of schizophrenia focuses on cognitive factors and to the extent that the characterization of such factors cannot fail to implicate our own reflexive analysis of what we mean by cognition (an analysis also posited under the same historicized circumstances), the diagnosis and, *a fortiori*, the treatment of schizophrenia cannot fail to exhibit an ineliminably ideological dimension. In particular, this is due to the normative import of the functional distinctions pertinent in schizophrenia, as well as to the horizonal and perspectived grasp of normative notions in general.

A third distinction follows readily enough: we cannot hope to provide a convincing disjunction of a principled sort between schizophrenic and mere schizoid-like properties within the terms of any viable society. Between diseased or disordered and normal functioning pertinent distinctions must always fall out along a continuum that is disjunctively sorted, for reasons that happen to be salient (but may change) within a particular self-examining society, however carefully (in a dialectical and objective sense) it may compare its own behavior with the range of behavior that another society exhibits.

These last three distinctions suggest some lines of inquiry for giving greater precision and coherence to our notion of schizophrenia. But they are not likely to alter the force of our principal findings.

References

Blanck, G. & Blanck, R. (1979). *Ego psychology II: Psychoanalytic developmental psychology*. New York: Columbia University Press.

Buchsbaum S. & Haler, R.J. (1987). Functions and anatomical brain imaging: Impact on schizophrenia research. *Special Report: Schizophrenia 1987*, 129-146. National Institute of Mental Health.

Foucault, M. (1977). *Discipline and punishment* (trans. Alan Sheridan). New York: Vintage Books.

Hamilton, N.G. (1988). *Self and others: Object relations therapy in practice*. New York: Jason Aronson.

Hempel, C.G. (1965). Fundamentals of taxonomy. In *Aspects of scientific explanation and other essays in the philosophy of science*. New York: Free Press.

Kuhn, T.S. (1970). *The structure of scientific revolutions*, 2nd ed. rev. Chicago: University of Chicago Press.

Margolis, J. (1966). *Psychotherapy and morality: A study of two concepts*. New York: Random House.

Margolis, J. (1986). *Pragmatism without foundations: Reconciling realism and relativism*. Oxford: Basil Blackwell.

Miller, D.R. & Jaques, E. (1988). Identifying madness: An interaction frame of reference. In H.J. O'Gorman (ed.), *Surveying social life*. Middletown, CT: Wesleyan University Press.

Shore, D. (Ed.), (1987). *Special Report: Schizophrenia 1987*. National Institute of Mental Health.

Rinsley, D. (1982). *Borderline and other self disorders*. New York: Jason Aronson.

Szasz, T.S. (1961). *The myth of mental illness*. New York: Harper Hoeber.

Wiener, M. (1989). Psychopathology reconsidered: Depressions interpreted as psychosocial transactions. *Clinical Psychology Review*, 9, 295-321.

10
Conceptualizations of Human Behavioral Breakdowns: An Analysis Using the Doctrine of Cultural Relativism

Horacio Fabrega, Jr.

Introduction

Anomalies in human social behavior that are not transient but sustained are phenomena that human groups have always had to contend with and explain. There are many ways in which such anomalies can be classified. One could use external- and observer-imposed conventions, or one could use those that are culturally specific and local to the society. Some anomalies may be judged positively by co-members; individuals who show these anomalies are likely to be valued and accorded power, status, and/or prestige. Other anomalies are disvalued and judged negatively. Whether or not the behaviors are judged as being willful is a further important consideration in the way behavioral anomalies are culturally defined.

Anomalies of behavior that are sustained and judged as not willful and negatively I term human behavioral breakdowns (HBB). These constitute the basic focus of this chapter. They are held to include all or some of the following: disturbances in mentation and awareness that render work and relationships unproductive, impairments in emotional well being, irregularities of social identity and conduct, and failures to meet standards of appearance, dress and cleanliness. A human behavioral breakdown encompasses behaviors that could be the object of professional psychiatric diagnoses as well as lay labels that might signify behavioral derangement or dilapidation. The term breakdown and/or disturbance means that the behaviors in question are defined as constituting a disruption in, or threat to, organized social life, and hence are generally disvalued.

The appearance that HBB possesses in a society has a cultural rationale. This means that the behaviors of the person showing HBB are (1) shaped and conditioned by culture and (2) labelled by co-members using conceptualizations and categories drawn from the culture. The society is held to possess a system of categories and explanatory frameworks by which sense is made of the self and the world, including HBB. In labelling a behavioral anomaly as an instantiation of HBB, a co-member of the culture has classified the behavior; he or she, in identifying it as a local variant of HBB, has "seen in it" criteria that make up the conceptual category HBB (as opposed to something else).

Although the label applied to HBB is by definition "negative," it does not follow that within a given society HBB are handled as medical problems. A fundamental issue in cultural psychiatry involves the question of what is medical in a society and culture, as opposed to what is moral, political, or religious, and on what bases these distinctions are made. This problem will not be addressed in this chapter. Societies are held to possess medical care "systems" which include illness theories, treatment schemes, locally produced or imported medical knowledge, practitioners and healers of different persuasion, institutions for training them, and social practices governing diagnosis, treatment, and prevention. It is in terms of these systems of knowledge and practice that people may diagnose and treat HBB as illness.

Emphasis on HBB as illness is important because, in general, labelling something an illness tends to bring into play special symbols, qualifications, and practices that have as their goal the restoration, amelioration, and assimilation of HBB (Parsons, 1951). Of course, this is not always possible. Some HBB that are labelled as illness may in fact be recurring, persistent, debilitating, and associated with increasing deterioration. This raises the important question of how the HBB come to be viewed and handled in the society in the event local treatment practices prove unavailing. It is implied that conventions about what constitutes HBB and adequate treatment may or may not be shared across societies and cultures: different societies or cultures may have different concepts of HBB—relationships between illness and HBB may also be different. In fact, the relationships between illness and HBB are likely to vary significantly across societies, within societies across time, and even within societies at one point in time but across social space (if the society is reasonably complex).

Human Behavioral Breakdowns in Different Societies and Eras

Ancient Near Eastern Societies

There exists very little in the way of information about conceptualizations of HBB in ancient Egyptian, Mesopotamian or Assyrian societies (Bark, 1988; Dawson, 1967; Jeste, et al., 1985; Kinnier Wilson, 1967; Saunders, 1963). Documents unearthed describe a relatively rich tradition of medicine consisting of elements that are mainly magical but sometimes rationalistic. It is thought that in Egyptian societies in particular, surgery was quite advanced. Some authors have concluded that people in Mesopotamian societies diagnosed phenomena resembling our psychoses, and dealt with these in terms of magical and ritual practices. Egyptian documents indicate that acute/confusional states were viewed as medical and handled as such. It is not possible to describe in detail characteristics of HBB and the manner in which they were explained and handled as social objects. Reports include general abstract behavioral descriptions that suggest HBB, for which treatment involving incantations was recommended. The phenomena in question are said to consist of "the verbatim utterances of certain schizophrenic patients who believe they were the center of a conspiracy" (Kinnier Wilson, 1967, p. 724) but the bases for these claims are not clear. Labels and explanatory frameworks about HBB are not available, and medical explanations about those HBB that were handled as illnesses are similar to explanations about other types of illnesses (e.g., illnesses of internal organs, surgical illnesses). Punishment by deities and/or demons and noxious material introduced into the body that produce decay are examples of "theories of illness" that have been described in relation to HBB.

Ancient Indian Societies

Ayurvedic Medicine constitutes one of the most elaborated systems of knowledge about human disease (Dube, 1978; 1985; Haldipur, 1984; Kutumbiah, 1969; Leslie, 1976; Obeysekere, 1977; Rao, 1975; Weiss, 1977). A complex physiology based on the humors (dosas), diet and nutrition, physical and social behavior, and relationship to the ecologic setting along with supernatural and metaphysical factors played a role in explanations of health, disease, and treatment. The Ayurvedic system is supremely philosophical, being an outcome of intricately elaborated notions involving the natural and immaterial as well as the mental and bodily. The system is said to be somatopsychic and psychosomatic, essentially endorsing an integrated holistic perspective about disease and health in which mental/psychological as well as bodily/physical/physiological factors are all implicated in diseases.

A great deal of material is available that describes instances of HBB in ancient Indian societies that were explained along medical lines. Observers indicate that insanity, madness and/or varieties of our "functional disorders" were identified and treated (Dube, 1978; Weiss, 1977). The etiology of these medicalized HBB was said to involve humoral alterations as well as spirit possession. Explanations encompassed psychological temperament, diet, environmental influences, and elaborate notions about the humors and organ functioning. Importantly, all illnesses—not just "psychiatric" ones—were explained in a similar fashion. In addition, this system of medicine appears to ascribe mental behavioral as well as bodily components to all illnesses, not just to HBB. In this sense, illnesses consisting of HBB were not sharply distinguished from other illnesses. However, it is notable that this theory describes HBB separately from other conditions. "The science of mental disease, or bhutuidya, occupies a major place in Atharva Veda. One of the eight chapters deals entirely with this subject" (Dube, 1978, p. 211). In the descriptions there is the tendency to abstract out of instances of HBB general indicators pertaining to thinking, emotion, and conduct that are inferable from social maladaptation. Dube (1978) says:

> In Ayurveda clinical syndromes are well described on the basis of behavioral symptoms alone (p. 224).

> A majority of the symptoms of different psychiatric illnesses reported in the Ayurvedic literature are behavioral, describing mental patients on the basis of observed symptomatology only (p. 226).

In this sense, the Indian concept of HBB was socio-psychological and adaptational. However, in contrast to what is known about the Near Eastern material, our knowledge of the Ayurvedic systems suggests the beginnings of an elaborated theory and typology about HBB, the components of which consist of descriptions of deviations in social and psychological behavior, and for which treatments were indicated.

A hallmark of Ayurvedic medicine could be said to be its functional or biographic/historical focus. Diseases involve disturbances in the person's whole being and are tailored to the individual. However, although a "functional view of disease" could be said to have been dominant, Ayurvedic medicine must be seen as also possessing features suggesting traces of an ontological view (this is particularly in evidence with respect to phenomena described earlier as HBB), because some disease entities appear to have been separately named and described. Ambiguity surrounds the concept of an ontological perspective on disease; some of these views merely require a general notion of contagion or seed that gives disease a separate identity; others the notion of a concrete, perhaps foreign, entity taking root in the body and featured by a natural history; while still others seem to admit that it would suffice to name and describe distinct types of illness possessed of an invariant profile of manifestations and course (Nutton, 1983; Pagel, 1972; Temkin, 1963). In this light, the term "unmãd" is used in Ayurvedic medicine to denote a type of HBB (insanity) whose features, in singling out psychological and social behavior changes (as well as bodily ones, to be sure), create a distinct category of illness. Moreover, renowned Indian physicians classified unmãd as an illness produced by bodily humors, mental humors, and their combination, and also as an illness involving supernatural possession and/or punishment that involves the entry of agencies and their removal for treatment. For example, Caraka describes a vata, itta, and kappa variety of unmãd (insanity) in accordance with the type of dosa (humor) implicated, and provides a syndromal description. Dube (1978) has equated Ayurvedic conceptions of HBB with DSM-III conceptions of psychiatric disorders. The correspondences that he draws in the pictures of HBB are rather general and involve abstracting parallel emphases about, and indicators of, medicalized HBB. Dube's material indicates that elaborated features of consciousness and psychologic experience were not singled out in the Indian system.

In summary, we observe in the medicine of ancient India an integrated somatopsychic view of disease that is elaborately functional (physiological, historical, and biographically contingent) and also, to a lesser extent, ontological. Importantly, the HBB singled out as unmãd and illness cannot be described as peculiarly mental, intellectualistic, or emotional, since all diseases partake of such phenomena as well as of bodily manifestations. No special emphasis seems to have been given to the course of unmãd in its classification. However, it should be emphasized that estimation of prognosis was crucial to the Ayurvedic physician (who graded seriousness in terms of his willingness to offer treatment) and that varieties of unmãd judged to result from a discordance of all three humors were recorded as dreadful and incurable, though whether diagnosis was rendered before the fact is not known.

Ancient Chinese Societies

The medicine of ancient China is distinctive because of its eclectic and syncretistic character (Agren, 1975; Chiu, 1981; 1986; Kleinman, 1975; Lin, 1981; Lu & Needham, 1980; Schiffeler, 1979; Tseng, 1973; Unschuld, 1983; Yanchi, 1988a, 1988b). Many theoretical schemes developed over the millennia and became prominent in different dynastic periods, only to recede as others occupied "center stage." Invariably, many borrowings and modifications took place among the various theoretical schemes or schools, so that ideas from different periods were never really eliminated but became incorporated (with or without modifications) in succeeding periods. It is thus difficult to establish clear conceptual boundaries between what once were more or less distinctive explanatory frameworks and theories. The latter were numerous and can be equated with the various ideo-logical/moralistic/religious traditions of China; namely, Confucianism, Taoism, and Buddhism, as well as with naturalistic/empirical traditions and demoniacal emphases that are deeply embedded in the history of the Chou dynasty. A dominant theoretical scheme was perhaps that described as systematic correspondence. This involved elaborate theories pertaining to the five phases and to Yin-Yang, which related an organ physiology, hierarchy among different organs, and circulation via conduits to dietary factors and environmental influences.

A distinguishing feature of "Chinese medicine" was the elaborated theoretical scheme in terms of which disease was explained, with the notion of balance and disharmony playing a critical role. A highly rational, systematic approach to diagnosis prevailed that aimed at inducing disturbed physiology as a means towards interpretation and empirical treatment. The imbalance or disharmony in inner bodily workings or in body-environment relatedness was realized in the form of a *symptom complex* which was the distinguishing marker of ill health, and was geared to the particularities of the individual. In other words, although symptoms constitute important units of explanation, diagnosis, and treatment, it is in their linkages and associations that one finds the essential ingredient of a condition of ill health. Such complexes (although subject to some description and codification) were related to the presenting picture of the person: "Chinese medicine does not distinguish different diseases; it differentiates symptom-complexes. A symptom complex is a complete summarization of the functioning of the body at a particular stage of illness" (Yanchi, 1988a, p. 18). A review of the theories of medicine of the ancient Chinese thus suggests that a functional and/or biographical/historical view of disease also prevailed.

Despite the dominance of a functionalist orientation, types of HBB were identified in ancient Chinese societies and given a measure of social specificity. Tseng (1973), for example, has been able to identify in ancient texts descriptions that conform to our "mental disorders." Chiu (1986) has pointed to the pitfalls of the view that in ancient China mental diseases existed as categorical/ontological entities, and emphasizes that, although suggestions of such a view seemed present in certain writings, the bulk of writings treat mental illness symptoms (along with other "physical" symptoms) as units of dysfunction that are explained in an integrated ethnophysiologic way. Distinctive symptom complexes for which herbs were prescribed frequently include behavioral changes found in our mental disorders. According to Unschuld (1983), behavioral disorders (having a specificity of some sort) were ascribed in some instances to excess mucus production in the heart. In the classic of Nan-Ching, madness is singled out as resulting from excess Yin influences in the Yin vessels. In Chinese texts forms of HBB described as madness/insanity are singled out but, characteristically, they are embedded in general descriptions about theoretical (Yin-Yang; Five Phase Theories; Organ Depots and channels) or practical (herbs for treatment of symptoms) issues that pertain to all conditions of ill health. In legal discussions about the matter of criminal responsibility, it is clear that madness as a distinct entity was given attention (Chiu, 1981). All of this suggests that HBB had a medically and socio-politically individuated character. This suggests that traces of an ontological view of illness were ascribed to HBB, but may have been less well elaborated than in the medicine of ancient India. The criteria of HBB viewed as madness are not entirely clear but it would appear that, as in India, general aspects of sociopsychological maladaptation (versus specific psychological aspects of mentation), were singled out.

Classical Mediterranean Societies

A great deal is known regarding how the people of the Greco-Roman period conceptualized aberrations and breakdowns of human behavior (Drabkin, 1974; Jackson, 1969, 1972; Moss, 1967; Rosen, 1968; Simon, 1978). Rosen (1968) has dealt with the general problem of conceptualization of HBB; namely, behaviors judged locally as odd, eccentric, and outright "mad." He points to the tradition early in antiquity of ascribing such behavior to supernatural causation (divine punishment). The problem of how behavioral anomalies are interpreted, which involves boundaries between normal and abnormal in the societies, is also discussed. For example, Rosen gives attention to evaluations of prophets that parallel those of Devereux (1956) regarding the shaman. He points out that not all HBB or forms of what an outside observer would describe as madness or schizophrenia were viewed as illnesses. It is very clear that behavioral anomalies and HBB phenomena, and their conceptualization (e.g., description, interpretation), were topics that were important to philosophers, play-rights and the populace. The roots of Western views of HBB can be traced to the general attitudes and interpretations prevalent in antiquity; this includes aspects of social labelling, stigmatization, and medicalization. Two things need to be singled out: (1) many instances of HBB were viewed as medical in nature; that is, conceptualized as illness; and (2) the medical texts of the Greeks and Romans used terminologies that are still with us today.

> The intact writings from ancient Greece and Rome, when they deal with the subject of mental disorders, tend to refer to three types of madness with sufficient regularity to suggest that they were well established as nosological categories ... these three traditional forms of madness—phrenitis, melancholia, mania—apparently had a certain descriptive constancy in the medical view of that era... (Jackson, 1969, p. 371).

The people of antiquity distinguished between acute and chronic forms of HBB. In the medical theory, HBB were regarded, along with other illnesses, as physiological disturbances (Jackson, 1969; 1973). The acute form, phrenitis (delirium), was associated with fever and referred to serious states of illness that either abated quickly or terminated in death. The chronic forms were variations of madness and have been associated with our principal functional psychiatric conditions. An important aspect of all of these conditions is that they were explained naturalistically and were dealt with like other illnesses. It would appear that the so-called chronic conditions were usually treated in the home with servants acting as custodians and "aides." The expectation was that these conditions would remit. How persons who were poor and showed HBB were handled is not clear. Rosen and others suggest that chronic, unremitted forms of HBB were common in public settings and were subject to scorn, ridicule, and fear because of their putative link to the supernatural and demonic.

Hallmarks of the theory of illness in the Classical and Hellenistic periods that historians of medicine single out as important are illustrated in the way the above mentioned forms of HBB were conceptualized (Nutton, 1983; 1984; 1985; Temkin, 1963). There existed a *functional* emphasis associated with the Hippocratic tradition and other schools. This view drew emphasis to disturbances in bodily and brain physiology; it was the uniqueness of the changes in light of the person's biography that constituted the illness. On the other hand, historians point to an *ontological* emphasis as well. In this instance, attention is drawn to the specificity, separateness, and alleged identity of a disorder (this topic is dealt with more fully below). With respect to symptoms one notes a complex assortment: intellectual functions including delusions and reality distortion are singled out but so are changes in emotional state, impulsiveness, violence, social indifference, and a number of general bodily symptoms. The variety of phenomena singled out as being criteria of medicalized forms of HBB in this period needs to be emphasized. The theories of personhood in classical Greece clearly drew on human reason, and conceptualizations of HBB figured importantly. In other words, madness/insanity also functioned as a symbol and metaphor that played a key role in conceptualizations of social order, morality, self-worth, and personal responsibility (Burkert, 1985; Simon, 1978). The conception of HBB as madness/insanity played a central role in philosophic and literary discussions. In the medical domain, however, purely psychological phenomena were not dominant, but rather were components of a range of behavioral and bodily symptoms that could accurately be described as integrated somato-psychically or holistically.

In summary, in the classical era conceptualizations of HBB as illness played an important cultural role in the society at large. What one could now describe as literary, political, religious, philosophic, and moral questions and pursuits were undertaken in terms of symbols about human reason and virtue that contrasted with phenomena intrinsic to medical varieties of HBB. In the strictly medical sphere, however, conceptualizations of HBB also drew emphasis to a range of phenomena that were non-psychologic in nature. Many of the items we today associate with schizophrenia were, in a general sense, intrinsic to these descriptions and conceptualizations of HBB, but in addition one finds references to a range of bodily and physiologic phenomena. In this sense, these medical conceptualizations are similar to those found in ancient India and China. To be sure, in these two societies, matters involving reason and morality played no less dominant a role. However, in the general cultural arena of India and China, symbols of the nature of HBB appear to have had less cultural play (although lack of availability of literature in English may cause this conclusion to be biased).

Smaller-Scaled Non-Western Societies

The basic criticisms pertaining to the universalistic claims of psychiatry in general, and with regards to topics such as schizophrenia in particular, have emanated from cultural anthropologists, and have been based on comparative work in smaller-scaled societies (Edgerton, 1969; Fabrega, 1974; 1989a; 1989b; 1989c; Murphy, 1976; Simons & Hughes, 1985). The nature and implications of these criticisms will be taken up later in this chapter. Suffice it to say for now that no one has ever asserted that a people are unacquainted with the phenomena we have labelled as HBB, which resemble, among other things, the phenomena that are currently labelled as schizophrenia. Instead, anthropological criticisms have been directed at basic assumptions about the essential nature of HBB; assumptions countered with observations involving such things as the relative incidence and prevalence of HBB, their varied manifest appearance, their varied interpretation, and—more recently—their varied course (Kleinman, 1988).

As formulated in this essay, HBB are not transitory or acute in nature but are extended in time. It is widely assumed that one reason why forms of HBB are not common in elementary societies is because of the differential survival of persons so afflicted. In subsistence economies, individuals functionally compromised with HBB cannot be expected to carry out their responsibilities, and are less likely to be maintained and kept alive. Another reason for the seemingly lower prevalence of HBB is said to be that the set of obligations and requirements inherent in smaller-scaled non-literate societies pose fewer social psychological demands on persons; in this instance, it is claimed, thus, HBB phenomena may be less likely to surface as social problems requiring special attention—medical or otherwise. Together with differing baselines and values regarding what constitutes HBB, this would contribute to spuriously low levels of HBB.

Important theoretical work in cultural psychiatry has involved the study of the local ("folk") criteria and interpretations of what had been described earlier as behavioral anomalies, as well as the study of HBB. It is not always the case that the behaviors in question are viewed as reflecting or indicating illness. Behaviors said to result from possession by spirits and even stereotyped syndromes can fail to be viewed and handled as illness. In many instances, however, HBB are equated with illness. A range of phenomena, encompassing social and psychological behavior (conduct, emotional dyscontrol, thinking) as well as an inability to participate and function in social life, are singled out by the people as indicators of a category that references medicalized HBB. In this sense, the criteria of HBB are also adaptational and draw on general socio-psychological norms, as in the "great traditions" of medicine described earlier.

The kinds of medical conceptualizations that people of smaller-scaled non-literate societies have demonstrated with respect to HBB are varied in nature. In general, depending on the society, HBB phenomena are ascribed to either natural causes (exposure to inclement weather), supernatural intervention (punishment from ancestors), or human malevolent doings (sorcery). There is no tendency for medicalized HBB to be equated with distinctive causal explanations across societies nor is there a tendency for it to be explained differently from other medical illnesses. There is perhaps a tendency for serious and/or chronic illnesses, regardless of their nature (psychiatric, medical) to be judged more dangerous, ominous, and threatening and to be explained in terms of supernatural and/or malevolent factors. An essential feature of the way illness, including some HBB, is handled in smaller-scaled societies is the social and public nature of diagnosis and curing. Illness constitutes a social and even political event in a group or village, and it brings into play moral and religious symbols. The unique social happenings in the group are incorporated in explanations of cause and activities of curing ceremonies and, together with details of the personal life of the person viewed as ill, come to be part of the social drama or spectacle of illness. The highly individuated nature of illness and its social basis argue against the existence of an ontological view of illness although illnesses do "exist" as named categories possessing a measure of symbolic specificity.

Preconditions of the Modern Concept of Schizophrenia

The concept of schizophrenia represents one of several medical concepts that have evolved in modern European societies to label occurrences of HBB. The concept owes its meaning to developments in the history of medicine in these societies. In short, the concept of schizophrenia is a modern European conception of HBB and, consequently, to understand it one must be provided with epistemological and ontological assumptions intrinsic to modern European medicine. An important development in the history of European medicine is the so-called "modern concept of disease."

It is, of course, very doubtful whether there can be said to exist one pervading or underlying concept of disease in contemporary science and medicine (Cohen, 1961; Pagel & Winder, 1968; 1972; Rather, 1959). Even in areas of medical discourse removed from psychiatry one can observe complexities and conflicts regarding essential features of disease. When one adds to this the quandaries devolving from mind/body and brain/behavior relations that come into play when theoretical elements of psychiatric disease are analyzed, a number of additional problems can be expected (Fabrega, 1975; 1980; Jackson, 1970; Riese, 1945; 1960). Thus, the discussion in this section needs to be evaluated with an appreciation of the many theoretical dilemmas attending any search for a modern concept of schizophrenia and disease in general.

There is disagreement about what exactly characterized the view of disease in antiquity and in the succeeding medieval period (which was dominantly influenced by it). A consensus is that the view of disease can be described as mainly functional in nature. In other words, characteristics of individuated sick persons, which were in turn explained by then prevailing physiologic ideas and theories, were of dominant importance. By "individuated," I mean that the circumstances of the person, such as diet, environment, psychological temperament, life style, astrological profile, and antecedent social conditions as well as humoral balances (constitutional and reactive to preceding factors) were all important in how a disease was explained and managed. Physicians very often were described as health advisors, since in promoting well-being and counteracting illness they used their knowledge of the biography of the whole person. Characterizing this functional view of disease, Pagel (1972), referring to Hippocratic writings, indicates that subtraction of what is in excess and addition of what is deficient was paramount: "...there is in fact only one disease, although its appearances vary with the places affected"— (p. 419). He goes on to add:

> In this concept, disease is determined by matter—something too much or something too little that is of the elements or the humors of their qualities. These or the way in which they are mixed, —complexion or temperament—or else their location are at fault and call for correction ... The *subject or essence of disease* is, therefore, *the diseased individual*. There are as many diseases as there are individuals. There is no disease, however, in its own right. There is no specific cause or development whereby one disease is specifically different from another (pp. 419-420).

In illuminating papers, Nutton (1983) and Temkin (1963) have put forth the idea that an ontological view of disease also existed in antiquity. In several instances, for example, Galen used the idea of "seeds of disease," which implies that disease has a separate identity and "plan" of its own with which it enters and lodges in the person, there to cause a series of changes. Furthermore, it has been pointed out that the vivid and compelling clinical descriptions of diseases in individuals are examples that approximate an ontological view insofar as such diseases are named and portrayed as abstracted clinical developments possessed of a temporal course. In short, classic descriptions of disease (those that, by our standards, provide an accurate depiction of clinical identity and course) presupposes a view that diseases have a "life of their own" —that is, an ontological view of disease. It would appear that this generalization about the medicine of antiquity, although valid, tends to weaken the idea that an exclusively functional perspective dominated. Perhaps one can conclude that an ontological perspective is implied in medical literature whereas in the actual practice of medicine the functionalist approach dominated.

The beginnings of a modern approach to disease have been traced to the writings of Paracelsus (1493-1541) and Van Helmont (1579-1644). Pagel (1972) is again particularly lucid in this regard.

> Paracelsus and Van Helmont agree that the ancient concept is wrong. They both believe that disease is a "thing" as real as any other object in nature. It does not lend itself to be impressed in terms of quality, mixture or displacement of something ... By contrast, disease to them has its own *specific seed.* It develops according to a plan intrinsic to its seed. It, therefore, requires a therapy radically different from rectifying excise or want. Instead, the specific seed must be removed or overcome by specific remedies (p. 420).

Many have discussed the changes in perspective about disease that have contributed to the "modern concept of disease." The writings of Harvey and Sydenham have been singled out together with those of Stahl, Hoffman, and Morgangni. In the 18th century, the writings of nosologists such as Cullen and Linneaus further elaborated the ontological perspective. Relying on ideas of mechanism, a number of general classifications of disease were developed based on considerations relating to the circulation of nervous and vital fluids, and propagation of nervous forces and energies. All of these developments eventually led to Virchow and the anatomoclinical view of the 19th century. Discoveries in the field of microbiology, of course, served to further concretize the ontological view that disease has an independent existence as well as its specific morbidity and natural history (Hudson, 1983).

A dominating ontological perspective with respect to disease thus seems rooted in academic and scientific developments of western European history. All of these developments may be considered to have created the conditions for a universalistic approach in which biological science plays a central role in the modern description and conceptualization of disease. By universalistic I mean to emphasize that diseases are held to be common to all of mankind. The same pathological changes, the same microbial agents, the same changes in metabolism, and the same interferences in function as well as symptoms can be held to affect the bodies of persons regardless of what they think, believe, and feel. In brief, a disease, in invading or transforming an individual's body, brings about a series of changes that parallel those produced in another regardless of the latter's cultural circumstances and peculiarities. Obviously, matters of immunological exposure, diet, and genetic structure need to be taken into account. The important point is that the modern concept of disease is ontological, which conditions a universalistic approach rooted in biological science. All of this is viewed as pancultural and serves to explain the phenomena of disease, irrespective of an individual's local culture.

In summary, the modern concept of disease rests on the philosophy of scientific objectivism. It is anchored in a position of biological reductionism, if not determinism. It allows one to identify and explain disease in all of mankind. Such a view points to underlying biological changes that operate panculturally; indeed, "underneath" culture. Conceptualizations of disease held in other societies and cultures or historical eras can be judged as being epiphenomenal to the correct biological conceptualization, which has been unsurpassed in its power to control and overcome the morbidity and mortality brought about by disease. It is the modern concept of disease, then, that allows an epidemiologist to confidently (and in a certain sense, correctly) claim that although certain persons in a non-Western society and culture are not viewed as sick, they are in fact diseased; and that those held to be sick with a cultural illness are in fact either biologically diseased or not really diseased at all.

Conceptualizations of HBB in 19th Century European Societies

During the 18th and especially 19th century the prevalence of HBB in European societies became increasingly a social problem. This topic has occupied social historians of psychiatry and cannot be gone into in detail here (Berrios & Hauser, 1988; Fabrega, 1989d; Scull, 1979).

Suffice it to say that with the political, economic, and social structural changes surrounding large scale urbanization, industrialization, and dependence on the market, the visibility, and perhaps incidence and prevalence, of HBB seemed to increase and became the concern of administrative agencies of the state. Initially (17th and 18th century) all classes of impoverished, socially marginal, dependent, and/or behaviorally impaired persons were placed in common institutions with little attention given to types of problems. There existed a "private trade" in forms of HBB termed lunacy, well documented for the 18th century, which largely provided for the confinement of those who were economically advantaged. During the 19th century, a number of social developments occurred including an increase in professional specialization, which resulted in the eventual emergence of psychiatry as a discipline. This led to the exploration of some forms of HBB as nsanity/madness (terms that were the object of new conceptualizations —see below); sufferers of HBB were placed in asylums and mental institutions. The social and cultural composition (including the language preference) of persons confined in these institutions had an effect on the kinds of conceptualizations of HBB that evolved, since these factors determined the type of patients proto-psychiatrists could interview directly and study (Berrios & Hauser, 1988).

Eighteenth century classifications of disease were general in nature and included HBB phenomena in such categories as the vesanias (Berrios, 1984; 1985; 1987a; 1987b; 1988a; 1988b; Bowman, 1975; Lopez-Pinero, 1983; Neuburger, 1945). Criteria for classification of these "species and genera" of illnesses involved "privileged features" in line with the principles of botanical systems. The categories formed were large and inclusive, being mainly descriptive and emphasizing intellectualistic features of insanity (e.g., the presence of prominent delusions) as well as behavioral disorganization. The nervous system (as indicated above) became a rubric for the explanation and classification of diseases in general including "entities" such as the vesanias. Diseases classified in this way, which at the time came to be termed neuroses, were thought of as organic (brain or nervous system) entities. Besides terms like insanity and madness, the term dementia was also used to categorize HBB phenomena. The latter was a descriptive term that had not yet acquired its association with pure cognitive deterioration, age, or reversibility.

Well before the 19th century, what we have termed HBB included phenomena that today we label or ascribe to organic factors. I am disregarding delirium ("phrenesy" in antiquity) since phenomena so labeled appear to have been limited to acute illnesses, whereas a hallmark of HBB is its temporal extension (sometimes permanent) and its all encompassing sociopsychological character; that is to say, its characterization of the total behavior of individuals not otherwise obviously physically ill. Early on, Celsus drew attention to the link between acute delirioid states that can leave a residue of true insanity which he in fact termed dementia. Berrios (1987a) quotes Willis to show that in the 17th century the concept of dementia was firmly linked to cognitive impairment and thus, by our standards, had acquired its present meaning. Moreover, the idea that cognitive impairment could be present since birth, and that this differed from its acquired forms, was well appreciated since the 17th century, according to Berrios. Neugebauer (1976) has shown that well before this period, deliberations in the Court of Livery involving the disposition of property of mentally compromised persons (i.e., showing HBB) were centrally concerned with the question of cognitive function and that "natural fools" constituted a category and referred to conditions judged separately from those of "lunatics," which no doubt included our dementias together with a range of other HBB phenomena (Neugebauer, 1976; 1979). Epilepsy was closely associated with that of dementia, delirium, and mental retardation in conceptualizations of HBB during the period preceding the 19th century. In fact, as is well known, the concept of epilepsy was central to the development of naturalistic medicine in antiquity and must be judged as being frequently applied to HBB phenomena throughout European history—in fact this is also the case in China and India (Temkin, 1971). By the 19th century, then, what we conceptualize as mental organic conditions each had their separate identity as concepts in the culture of medicine and in the society at large, and all were part of general conceptualizations of HBB. During the 19th century, many of these concepts were more clearly separated from other conceptualizations of HBB, and eventually became integrated within the discipline of neurology.

Developments in the conceptualization of medical forms of HBB during the 19th century that fall squarely within the psychiatric tradition have been well described. Altschule (1976a; 1976b) has provided documentation of the thinking of Crichton (on looseness of thinking), Pinel (on an extended view of dementia as cognitive impairment), Haslam (on "hebephrenic" disorders of puberty), and many others. Berrios and Hauser (1988) drew attention to the influential role that Kahlbaum had on Kraepelin in emphasizing natural history and course, as well as underlying "essential" aspects (as opposed to "surface" presentations) of any behavioral disorder that could explain HBB. In other words, emphasis came to be placed on the underlying process of development and course of mental diseases rather than surface symptomatic characteristics.

By the late 19th century, as a result of scientific efforts of various proto-psychiatrists and, in conjunction with the efforts of Kraepelin, a modern conceptualization of many forms of HBB had developed that involved an elaboration and transformation of the older view. The older view included the following: (1) many HBB are medical in nature; (2) medical HBB can be placed in different categories such as insanity/madness/lunacy viewed purely as intellectual or social psychological incapacity; dementia, a subset of the preceding and concentrating heavily on cognitive impairment; and mental incapacity that was congenital (natural fools); and (3) the categories of HBB are largely descriptive, functional, and based on symptoms and presumed global "nervous system" dysfunction. The newer view emphasized the possibility of distinctive disease entities, each of which had a putative identity that included cause, essential mechanism or lesion in the nervous system, and temporal profile.

A key late 19th century development, besides the modern concept of mental disease entities, was the formation of a descriptive language of psychopathology (Berrios, 1985). Whereas 18th and early 19th century descriptions of insanity had been global and social-psychological (in this way very similar to descriptions in other medical systems such as Ayurveda), the new semiology of psychopathology concerned itself with the development of categories pertaining to purely psychological phenomena. Thus, forms of cognition, perception, volition, emotion, and mental experience in general, became the objects of analysis. Complementing a richer conceptualization of HBB involving discrete disease entities was a richer conceptualization about how these entities might manifest themselves in behavior and adaptation.

In discussing the evolution of the concept of schizophrenia, Altschule (1976a; 1976b) has indicated that the idea of specific etiologies was a 19th century development, being associated with developments in pathological anatomy, microbiology, and toxicology. In earlier periods, there was

> nowhere in medicine any conviction concerning specific etiologies for any diseases. Hence, the etiology of mental diseases was the same as for all others, i.e., psychological factors, environmental factors, and humoral factors. All diseases were in effect no more than syndromes, and this applied also to mental disorders. (Altschule, 1976a)

In the 19th century, then, new ideas about causation that strengthened the view of diseases as naturalistic objects (ontology of disease) were borrowed from general medicine and began to be applied to what we have termed HBB. Many of the categories of disease in the disciplines of neurology and psychiatry serve to explain certain varieties of HBB in contemporary medicine and society. Here I am mainly concerned with schizophrenia, which is viewed as the most important modern conceptualization of HBB. This phase of European conceptualizations of HBB is well known, amply documented and alive in contemporary research; there is no need to review it here (Berrios, 1987c; Hoenig, 1982; 1983; Scharfetter, 1975).

Two Approaches to the Study of Schizophrenia in Relation To Culture

In 1956 George Devereux wrote an influential article entitled "Normal and abnormal: The key problem of psychiatric anthropology." In his article he discussed the grounds on which one could qualify behavioral phenomena in a particular culture as psychopathological, as opposed to healthy and adaptive. Devereux's reasoning pushed a key problem of cultural psychiatry into the intrapsychic sphere, there to be unravelled by careful assessments of how psychological conflicts were structured. He acknowledged the centrality of social and cultural factors by emphasizing that psychological conflicts were culturally contextualized and shaped, and that, moreover, the behavioral expressions of those conflicts were interpreted in terms of cultural conventions. His analysis was centered on the mode of adjustment of whole persons; he used as an example the shaman whose behavior could appear erratic, schizophrenic, dissociated, etc., since it involved constant intercourse with the supernatural and entailed personalized misinterpretations of reality. A prototypical question was the following: was the shaman normal or was he instead "really" schizophrenic but merely labelled differently, being "protected" by a role that sanctioned "pathological" experiences? Devereux's logic was consistent with that of Silverman (1967), who presented a rationale for how an acute schizophrenic syndrome, when played out in a local culture, could come to transform a person's mode of thinking and identity (by the unfolding of schizophrenia in the light of cultural meanings) so as to lead to the career of a shaman.

In Devereux's (1956) formulation, psychopathology consisted in the playing out of culturally specific conflicts that are common in the culture but ordinarily not problematic in the minds of other co-members. Such conflicts were said to be located in the individual's ethnic unconscious. The marginality of the role selected by the shaman was said to constitute one indicator of psychopathology, since it locates him or her in a position that is deviant and hence discrediting and potentially mortifying. Moreover, because it requires the shaman to continually play out the culturally specific conflicts, it unduly burdens him or her and closes off opportunities for psychological growth, development, and autonomy in the society. Another indicator of the psychopathology of the shaman was said to reside in the stability and patterning of the psychological defenses that were relied on to resolve the conflicts of the ethnic unconscious. Such defenses were assumed to be either weak or insufficient to protect the shaman from behavioral difficulties. Devereux indicated that this can also be dramatically shown at later stages in the life of the shaman. Normal persons of the culture, who by definition harbor similar ethnic unconscious conflicts, have presumably developed stronger and more flexible psychological defenses that are protective and that negate the behavioral difficulties devolving from these conflicts.

In the Devereux (1956) formulation, constituent symptoms of psychopathology do not receive primary attention. Such things as delusions, hallucinations, or other elements of psychopathology are not addressed directly, and when they are, they are looked at in psychoanalytic terms and in relation to intracultural or idiosyncratic conflicts, all examined in terms of the metapsychology of psychoanalysis. This formulation stipulates a version of cultural relativism with respect to psychiatric illness since it acknowledges cultural differences in the way behavioral anomalies and/or possible HBB might be labelled and played out, but argues that psychiatric illness (e.g., schizophrenia) is a universal sort of thing that can be reliably measured and diagnosed cross culturally; in this instance using the universalistic language of psychoanalysis. Even this version of cultural relativism is judged problematic by Murphy (1976) who in arguing against the labelling perspective of psychiatric illness emphasizes strong universalistic aspects of schizophrenia; in particular, that schizophrenic behavior looks the same and, more importantly, tends to be judged similarly in different cultures (Alaska and Africa). Murphy's paper gave momentum to a universalist perspective on psychiatric illness and, together with the ascendancy of neurobiology, has achieved dominance in American psychiatry. An analysis of this position and related ones is taken up below.

An important feature of Devereux's formulation is that psychotic behavior is held to possess a culturally distinctive rationale and form. Culture creates distinctive stresses, and can provide models or standardized forms of psychotic behavior to which sick persons conform. Even when these standardized behaviors are not in evidence, an important element of the behavior of the psychotic person involves (the misuse of) cultural symbols and cultural ways of thinking, feeling, and behaving that render the behavior comprehensible even if psychotic. From the standpoint of diagnosis, however, the content of behavior is secondary; it is how this content is constructed and patterned that determines the diagnosis of abnormality or psychosis. Devereux contrasts the (sick) behavior of shamans and of persons showing ethnopsychoses (culture-bound syndromes) with the behavior of "ordinary psychotics." In summary, in this theory of schizophrenia or abnormality, the content of behavior provides data that an examiner uses in order to reach a diagnosis. He or she does so, however, by evaluating it in terms of forms or structures based on psychoanalysis and an understanding of culture.

The Devereux formulation regarding the nature of psychosis and schizophrenia with its psychodynamic formulations expunged is not inconsistent with the dominant approach in contemporary psychiatry that gives emphasis to the form rather than the content of a syndrome of behavior. In this latter approach little emphasis is given to the question of whether a putatively schizophrenic person is judged locally as normal or abnormal, for it is the behavioral syndrome that constitutes the analytic unit, not a person's mode of general adjustment in his or her culture (Devereux's unit of analysis). The important question is whether a particular cultural syndrome of behavior displays a difference in form or structure when compared to an allegedly similar syndrome seen in another culture. More specifically, is a cultural variety of HBB different in form (structure) from schizophrenia as stipulated in biomedical psychiatry?

Implicit in the form versus content paradigm is the notion that there exists a universal mode of psychological experience and that, as a consequence, any clinically relevant syndrome of behavior can be said to reflect a common underlying pattern, architecture, or taxon of behavior. All of the forms of behavioral syndromes or illnesses of mankind, it is assumed, can be reduced to, or conform to, a finite set of taxa such as schizophrenia, bipolar disease, anxiety, startle reactions, and acute/agitated panic attacks. Superficial cross cultural differences in these behavioral syndromes are to be expected insofar as persons may hold different beliefs about self and reality, and may have different ways of conceptualizing and displaying mental experiences, and different ways of behaving in relation to a behavioral environment that differs as a function of culture. However, differences in the content of experience or behavior are held to be trivial; it is the underlying form that is salient. It is assumed that this underlying form is conditioned by human evolution and, hence, is culturally invariant, constituting as it were the psychic unity of mankind.

The form-versus-content paradigm has been lucidly stated by Jaspers in 1963:

> Form must be kept distinct from content which may change from time to time, e.g., the fact of a hallucination is to be distinguished from its content, whether this is a man or a tree ... Perceptions, ideas, judgments, feelings, drives, self-awareness, are all forms of psychic phenomena: they denote the particular mode of existence in which content is presented to us. It is true, in describing concrete psychic events we take into account the particular content of the individual psyche, but from the phenomenological point of view it is only the form that interests us ... (pp. 58-59) (quoted in Berrios, 1988b, p. 32).

The position of Schneider is equally clear:

> Diagnosis looks for the "how" (form) not for the "what" (the theme or content). When I find thought withdrawal, then this is important to me as a mode of inner experience and as a diagnostic hint, but it is not of diagnostic significance whether it is the devil, the girlfriend or a political leader who withdraws the thoughts. Wherever one focuses on such contents diagnostics recedes: one sees then only the biographical aspects or the existence open to interpretation (quoted in Hoenig, 1982, p. 396).

The thesis involving form versus content includes the following: (1) there exists a pancultural/panhuman form or structure to psychological experience; (2) this structure or form is given by the discoveries of the nineteenth century involving the phenomenology of experience; to the effect that awareness consists of distinctive categories, such as beliefs, judgments, perceptions, volitions/intentions, feelings/emotions, etc.; (3) such categories are like modes of awareness or modes of experience that characterize a conscious person at any point in time and across time; (4) such categories account for, indeed constrain and structure, the experience of self and reality, and underlie or regulate ongoing behavior; (5) disruptions of these categories of experience are realized in a person's awareness, sense of self, and behavior; (6) such disruptions constitute psychopathology; and (7) the categories, structures, or forms of psychopathology are universal, since they reflect disturbances in the universal normal pattern in which human experiences are cast.

The form-versus-content approach seems geared to looking at behavior as culturally decontextualized. The meanings of the content of behavior are ignored and the structure or form is all important. Moreover, the claim that a cultural variety of HBB or "schizophrenia" actually involves a difference in the form of schizophrenia as stipulated in Western biomedical psychiatry would appear inconsistent: Schizophrenia structures do not vary as a function of culture, for "culture" is equivalent to "content," which is irrelevant for diagnosis. In contrast, the approach of Devereux requires the analyst to look at behavior in cultural terms. On the other hand, the litmus test in the Devereux (1956) approach is the architecture of the behavior looked at, not only intrapsychically, but also in relation to the way the culture programs individuals. Culture, in other words, is not only responsible for the surface or content of behavior but also for part of its structure; that is, the nature of the conflicts, stresses, and the patterning of psychological defenses brought to bear on them. When an item of behavior or a putative syndrome is shown to reflect a faulty architecture, it is diagnosed as abnormal or psychotic. Here, although the analyst is required to take culture and content seriously, it is still in terms of how normality is held to be structured intrapsychically as stipulated in an external theoretical schema (psychoanalytic theory) that determines the diagnosis. In the Devereux paradigm, then, there exist culturally distinctive psychopathological structures (looked at psychoanalytically), whereas in the form versus content paradigm there exists only one common form that reflects psychosis panculturally.

The Weak Form of the Doctrine of Cultural Relativism in Relation to the Concept of Schizophrenia

The weak form of cultural relativism (Spiro, 1986) points to the existence of variability in social psychological characteristics of man, but acknowledges that cultures also display *universal features* since cultural diversity is constrained or limited by adaptive evolutionary imperatives. This view holds that many of the social and psychological characteristics of man are a response to (in addition to differences in culture), a set of species-specific needs and hence determined by biological, ecological, and social (e.g., socialization practices, exigencies of group living) factors. The social and psychological universals posited amount to a view about the *psychic unity of man* and would be easily accommodated to our understanding of the concept of schizophrenia and the behavioral entity that is denoted by it.

A cultural relativist holding this position could claim that the contemporary view about schizophrenia applies to all of mankind provided one takes into account problems in linguistic translation.

Schizophrenia is rooted in genetic structures, and is the product of (or can be characterized by) distinctive neurophysiologic and neurochemical processes or changes (e.g., smooth pursuit eye movements). It is realized in rather distinctive social and psychological behaviors (e.g., social deterioration, delusions, hallucinations, first rank symptoms, and impairment in monitoring of willful actions). The appearance of the illness may look slightly different cross culturally, but its form or structure could be shown to be universal, once cultural and linguistic differences are taken into account. This view relies on concepts such as pathoplasty and form versus content (see above) which allow for content or "surface differences" in schizophrenia but stipulate commonalities in structure or form.

Differences in the social consequences of schizophrenia cross-culturally are a definite anomaly for the position of weak cultural relativism. How an occurrence of schizophrenia is interpreted and its social trajectory depend largely if not exclusively on such things as differences in biological factors (e.g., degree of severity), psychological factors (e.g., intelligence), and social factors (e.g., economic status, education); but not, it would appear, on local cultural meanings, since schizophrenia is always disvalued (i.e., seen as HBB) and labelled medically (Murphy, 1976). If local medical interpretations of HBB significantly mitigate the stress produced in the family environment by the expressed emotion directed at the schizophrenic, then positing an influence of culture on the course of illness can be justified.

A weak cultural relativist would see little problem in the claim that it is meaningful and fruitful to regard schizophrenics as ill regardless of how they may be viewed in a culture. Moreover, their apparent claim is, that schizophrenics are in fact universally recognized as ill regardless of cultural differences (Murphy, 1976). Someone who is a shaman and (by external standards) eccentric or disordered, suffering from what we termed earlier "behavioral anomalies," would most likely not be presumed to show schizophrenia. That such a person might be judged as normal (or "super-normal") would be seen as reflecting a cultural naivete due to imperfect knowledge or frank irrationality. The argument regarding what is a rational or valid belief even applies, in principle, intraculturally: clinicians frequently diagnose patients who deny that they are in any way ill; they also claim that a particular person's interpretation that his cancer results from witchcraft is irrational. This highlights the link between cultural relativism and the problems of rationality in general: can one claim, (and if so, on what grounds), that some beliefs are true and valid whereas others which are irrational? This question raises a number of theoretical issues that cannot be pursued here (Hollis & Lukes, 1982; Wilson, 1970). Implicit in the thinking of the weak cultural relativist is that biomedical theories are more powerful, allow better prediction and control, and provide better descriptions and explanations generally about human psychological and social regularities.

In summary, regardless of whether one refers to the schizophrenia concept or the schizophrenia entity (i.e., the "disease" itself), a weak cultural relativist is little troubled by the study of schizophrenia in relation to culture. In the weak form of the doctrine of cultural relativism much of the theory and knowledge pertaining to schizophrenia and its application to all human societies regardless of culture is accepted as veridical and appropriate. This perspective thus encourages scientific research aimed towards developing pancultural (universal) generalizations about schizophrenia.

The Strong Form of the Doctrine of Cultural Relativism and Its Relation to Schizophrenia

The Schizophrenia Concept

One who believes in a strong form of cultural relativism would regard universalist claims about the concept of schizophrenia as problematic, if not impermissible. Descriptive propositions about the nature of the world (e.g., pertaining to who is schizophrenic), as well as evaluative ones (our theory of HBB is better than earlier ones or that of a nonliterate society's), would be viewed as conditioned by, and relative to, the ways of life and standards of a particular group, culture, or individual. The shaman in question, in other words, is viewed as normal and effective in the society in question and not as ill or defective, as schizophrenics or hysterics are described in Western societies, and, indeed, as others in the local society may be described who do receive culturally specific labels of sickness. Hence, he or she should not be diagnosed or labeled as schizophrenic for in the culture/society they are not only not viewed as ill, but are considered resourceful and accorded prestige. In brief, the strong cultural relativist holds as axiomatic the position of *normative relativism* to the effect that there are no legitimate transcultural standards with which to compare descriptive or evaluative propositions, or social and psychological characteristics found in different cultures/societies. In this version of cultural relativism, all cultural objects and theories are viewed as conditioned by local conventions, meanings, and social institutions. Moreover, such objects and theories are of equal worth in a descriptive and moral sense. For example, the aims of a medical system in a non-literate society are different from those of our society. It is with respect to those culturally specific aims that local concepts and theories of medicine and their approaches to treatment of locally defined illnesses should be judged; our disease terms and our aims of cure, eradication, or morbidity should not be the standards for judgment (Fabrega, 1976).

The Schizophrenia Entity

Exponents of the strong form of cultural relativism hold that some of the social and psychological properties that are said by Western researchers to be characteristic of schizophrenia would apply to schizophrenics everywhere regardless of how they might be characterized (e.g., as shamans) in the local culture. They see fundamental changes in perception, cognition, and the overall sense of reality and of self as intrinsic and universal alterations in biological and socio-psychologic characteristics produced by the genetically conditioned "lesion" of schizophrenia. Here, then, they would be describing these alleged characteristics of schizophrenia as partly neuropsychologic; that is, placing them near the physiologic level, and seeing them as direct outcomes of neuroanatomic and neurophysiologic alterations. (These views pertaining to the physiology and/or neurochemistry of schizophrenia are clearly held by the weak cultural relativist and might also be held by the "radical" cultural relativist—see below.) In the logic of a strong cultural relativist, these sorts of characteristics, if they do prove to be pancultural, would be explained as outcomes of the universal culture pattern and the psychic unity of mankind (which is denied by the "radical" cultural relativist).

While acknowledging on scientific grounds the power, value, and universality of the biomedical theory of schizophrenia, a strong cultural relativist is reluctant to apply and use indiscriminately the knowledge of psychiatry in a socially descriptive and/or evaluative sense—for an example, to deal with schizophrenia as a social problem without a cultural warrant or approval. In the logic of a relativist sociology of knowledge, claims about "physiologic" characteristics of schizophrenia are examples of what passes as "evidencing reasons" in the causal theories produced by physiologists and psychologists. All of this is seen as having little or nothing to do with "institutionalized patterns of knowledge," and is considered hardly relevant for an understanding of "reason in action" (Barnes & Bloor, 1982).

Strong cultural relativists accept that schizophrenia has physiologic properties but still allow for cultural influences on its form. They see such things as the first rank symptoms as psychologic changes determined by local (i.e., Western) concepts pertaining to reality and personhood, and not as changes that are universal or biological (Fabrega, 1989c). They would thus judge some of the enterprise of psychiatric transcultural epidemiology as narrowly conceived, if not misguided. Narrowly conceived because descriptive propositions about Western schizophrenics are used to select indicators of the putatively real and universal schizophrenia illness. Such indicators of symptoms could be seen as conditioned by Western culture and psychology, and important because of emphases peculiar to that culture. In other words, only characteristics of Western schizophrenia are used as the model to study other non-Western schizophrenias, whereas an open (not closed) conception about the social and psychological characteristics of schizophrenia should be used as a guide for cross-cultural research. A strong relativist would also claim that the course of even a physiologically conceived schizophrenia is importantly influenced by the cultural nature of the social psychological characteristics of schizophrenia and by the cultural nature of the social responses to the person showing them. In other words, more than just variations in associated conditions of a schizophrenic episode (severity, social status, intelligence, the assumptions of the weak cultural relativist pertaining to possible differences in course) would account for differences in schizophrenias cross culturally. For the strong cultural relativist, ethnopsychologic structures and social labelling responses (i.e., cultural phenomena) are assumed to influence the "biologic" unfolding of schizophrenia (Fabrega, 1989c; Kleinman, 1988).

In summary, exponents of the strong form of cultural relativism accept descriptive and evaluative propositions about the *biomedical* character of schizophrenia (i.e., its physiology) but not its social medical character. They allow for the possibility that culture can have a more powerful role in "programming" the brain. This would have the effect that distinctive selves and modes of defining self and reality would condition social psychologic characteristics of schizophrenia (Fabrega, 1989a; b; c). Some of these characteristics, possibly the first rank symptoms and other characteristics heavily conditioned by Western psychologic and dualistic assumptions, would be judged as culturally determined and not biologically determined (universal or pancultural). The reports of clinicians and social science researchers of the universality of symptoms would be dismissed mainly on empirical grounds (the failure to adopt an ethnopsychologic frame of reference, the quandaries of translating across language and cultural communities). Overriding such differences as to phenomenology and perhaps course of schizophrenia are agreements about the many other parameters of schizophrenia that a strong cultural relativist would share with the weak cultural relativist, for both persons subscribe to the tenets of scientific objectivism, as these pertain to most of the universal generalizations about schizophrenia. Needless to say, the strong cultural relativist welcomes cross cultural research in psychiatry as legitimate and useful (Kleinman, 1988).

The Radical Form of the Doctrine of Cultural Relativism and Its Relation to Schizophrenia

Persons who subscribe to what Spiro (1986) terms the strong form of cultural relativism, a position he describes as epistemological relativism, are here termed radical cultural relativists. This position seems more neatly profiled. It views cultures as constituting ways of thinking, feeling, and behaving that are so different as to be incommensurable. Moreover, its exponents would appear to view the task of the social sciences as that of *interpreting* and not explaining or comparing the way cultures work. Thus, the influence of cultures is seen as so pervasive that it renders either vacuous or non-tenable ideas such as the psychic unity of man and the possibility of meaningful cross-cultural comparison. In conjunction with wholesale cultural determinism, one finds a notion of the maximal degree of cultural variability or diversity, which overrides the possibility of any meaningful pancultural generalizations involving social and cultural characteristics of man.

With respect to schizophrenia, a radical cultural relativist would hold that cultural influences are so pervasive, and the differences between cultures so extensive, that it makes little sense to treat as comparable (much less as equivalent) Western concepts and the syndrome of schizophrenia, on the one hand, and non-Western conceptualizations and putative syndromes subsumed by HBB on the other. He or she would claim that much, if not all, of biomedical psychiatry is best viewed as describing purely physiologic phenomena and hence as falling outside the domain of human symbolic behavior, the proper domain of the social sciences. To the extent that biomedical descriptions of schizophrenia address social and psychological characteristics, including symbolic behavior, it would be seen as having little warrant as an explanatory system in other non-Western cultures and societies. This is so because biomedical psychiatry is geared to, and based on, western European cultural conceptions of man and social order.

Implicit in the position of radical cultural relativism appears to be the notion that the disciplines of psychiatry and psychology, as an example, constitute a Western psychiatry and psychology. In other words, these disciplines serve to describe and explain social and psychologic behavioral phenomena as realized in Western European and Anglo-American societies. It seems appropriate here to mention the presuppositions associated with the emerging field of cultural psychology:

> A social-cultural environment is an intentional world. It is an 'intentional' world because its existence is real, factual and forceful, but only as long as there exists a community of persons whose beliefs, desires, emotions, purposes and other mental representations were directed at it, and are, thereby, influenced by it ... Intentional worlds are human artifactual worlds, populated with products of our own design ... Such intentional ... things exist only in intentional worlds ... [and] such things would not exist independent of our involvements with them and reactions to them; and they exercise their influence in our lives because of our conceptions of them (Shweder, 1990, p. 2).

In this view, "schizophrenia" would seem to constitute an intentional object or thing—a thing apparently made, bred, fashioned, fabricated, invented, designated, and constituted by Western biomedical science. To be sure, the view that Western concepts of psychosis and schizophrenia are created for special purposes that are culturally and historically contingent, and that biomedical psychiatry may not have real or appropriate application in other cultural settings because these are governed by alternative epistemologies, is consistent with the view identified earlier as strong cultural relativism. It is the use to which Western biomedical psychiatry is put and the possibility of drawing useful knowledge from truly comparative cross cultural studies that distinguish the radical form of cultural relativism.

The statement that schizophrenia is an intentional object has many layers of meaning. In the most trivial sense, it simply means that the label and syndrome have been fashioned by special disciplines for their own purposes. Both label and concept are created to help eliminate HBB through treatment and thereby validate the respective disciplines in the society. In a deeper sense, the intentionality of schizophrenia means that broad ranging Western cultural epistemologies (affecting ethnotheories of emotion, persons, modes of thinking and perceiving, etc.) are linked to the schizophrenia concept and syndrome, and that they shape and condition the mode of cognition, perception, and behavior in a very encompassing way.

Consequently, when a possible disturbance compromises the neuro-organic machinery of the brain, the result is a schizophrenic illness as culturally shaped and defined in Western and Anglo-American societies. If indeed a universal neurobiologic lesion of "schizophrenia" exists, the effect of cultural differences will be the production of behavioral changes that may or may not be realized as behavioral anomalies, HBB, or illness. It is, of course, possible that radical cultural relativists may subscribe to a radical form of the social labelling theory in which schizophrenia is seen purely as a product of social attributions. Finally, since Western biological science is seen as integral to the biomedical enterprise and both are seen as constituting a highly individualistic (as opposed to socialized) ideology of medicine that unduly naturalizes and beclouds human predicaments surrounding sickness, it would seem that the position of radical cultural relativism is highly consistent with some of the ideas of critical theorists of the Frankfurt school, and indeed with those of critical medical anthropologists regarding the enterprise of natural science and biomedicine (Geuss, 1981; Schepper-Hughes & Lock, 1986).

Persons who subscribe to a radical form of cultural relativism not only hold that the epistemology of one society or culture cannot be equated, compared, or analyzed with respect to another but also believe that the enterprise of a universal biological and social science cannot be meaningfully sustained. They would hold that only trivial or vacuous generalizations about society and behavior can be asserted (e.g., all people have local views of what is normal versus abnormal, what is illness versus health, what is a delusion versus a belief). They would hold, for example, that meaningful generalizations or theories about the historical and cultural ubiquity of concepts and phenomena subsumed under HBB are not possible. The claim that other people's concepts of HBB map or code what our concept of schizophrenia maps or codes, or that their shamans are really our schizophrenics, would be judged as gross simplifications of the meaning of cultural objects. To defend their position they would point to the numerous ways in which cultural objects and claims about them connect to the epistemology and perspective of a people; they would also mention the incommensurability of these cultural epistemologies. Ultimately, radical cultural relativists would assert the impossibility or misguided nature of a universal science about persons and behavior, and possibly that the ultimately materialistic bases of Western political economic claims about man are wrapped in the cloaks of biomedical and medical/psychological science.

In radical cultural relativism, schizophrenia seems eliminated as a concept or syndrome that is relevant to alternative societies and cultures. These constitute "incommensurable" intentional worlds with their own Japanese, Indian, or Chinese HBB syndromes and culturally based conceptualizations. The radical form of the theory of cultural relativism thus runs counter to the basic presuppositions of biomedicine, public health, and mental health policy, which are grounded in scientific objectivism.

Moreover, the theory would seem to contain some very problematic implications. As an example, criticisms and deliberations by professional bodies about the misuses of the schizophrenia concept by Soviet psychiatrists and allied social political personnel would presumably be seen as inappropriate and misinformed. Such criticisms would be seen as premised on the European/Anglo-American intentional world of HBB where the schizophrenia concept belongs and not applicable to the intentional Soviet world where an incommensurable language and culture predicate an altogether different conceptualization and approach to HBB phenomena. Alternatively, they would see differences in the way the schizophrenia concept is used as illustrating the essentially political and cultural character of our allegedly neutral and objectivist science.

References

Agren, H. (1975). A new approach to Chinese traditional medicine. *American Journal of Chinese Medicine, 3*(3), 207-212.

Altschule, M.D. (1976a). Historical perspective - evolution of the concept of schizophrenia. In S. Wolf and B.B. Berle (Eds.), *The biology of the schizophrenic process*, pp. 1-15. New York: Plenum.

Altschule, M.D. (1976b). *The development of traditional psychopathology*, pp. 1-14. New York: Wiley & Sons.

Bark, Nigel M. (1988). On the history of schizophrenia. *New York State Journal of Medicine, 88*, 374-383.

Barnes, B. & Bloor, D. (1982). Relativism, rationalism and the sociology of knowledge. In M. Holis and S. Lukes (Eds.), *Rationality and relativism*, pp. 21-47. Cambridge: Massachusetts Institute of Technology Press.

Berrios, G.E. (1984). The psychopathology of affectivity: conceptual and historical aspects. *Psychological Medicine, 14*, 303-313.

Berrios, G.E. (1985). Descriptive psychopathology: conceptual and historical aspects. *Psychological Medicine, 15*, 745-758.

Berrios, G.E. (1987a). Dementia during the seventeenth and eighteenth centuries: a conceptual history. *Psychological Medicine, 17*, 829-837.

Berrios, G.E. (1987b). Historical aspects of psychoses: 19th century issues. *British Medical Bulletin, 43*(3), 484-498.

Berrios, G.E. (1987c). The fundamental symptoms of dementia praecox or the group of schizophrenias. In C. Thompson (Ed.), *The origins of modern psychiatry*, pp. 200-209. Chichester: Wiley & Sons.

Berrios, G.E. (1988a). Melancholia and depression during the 19th century: a conceptual history. *British Journal of Psychiatry, 153*, 298-304.

Berrios, G.E. (1988b). Historical background to abnormal psychology. In E. Miller and P.J. Cooper, (Eds.), *Adult abnormal psychology*, pp. 26-51. New York: Churchill Livingstone.

Berrios, G.E. & Hauser, R. (1988). The early development of Kraepelin's idea on classification: a conceptual history. *Psychological Medicine, 18*, 813-821.

Bowman, I.A. *William Cullen (1710-90) and the primacy of the nervous system.* (1975). (Ph.D. Dissertation) Indiana: Indiana University.

Burkert, W. (1985). *Greek religion.* Cambridge: Harvard University Press.

Chiu, M.L. (1981). Insanity in imperial China. In A. Kleinman and T.Y. Lin, (Eds.), *Normal and abnormal behavior in Chinese culture*, pp. 75-94. Reidel: Dordrecht.

Chiu, M.L. (1986). *Mind, body and illness in a Chinese medical tradition* (Ph.D. Dissertation), Cambridge: Harvard University.

Cohen, H. (1961). The evolution of the concept of disease. In B. Lush, (Ed.), *Concepts of medicine, pp. 159-169.* New York: Pergamon Press.

Dawson, W.R. (1967). The Egyptian medical papyri. In D. Brothwell and A.T. Sandison, (Eds.), *Diseases in Antiquity.* Illinois: CC Thomas.

Devereux, G. (1956). Normal and abnormal: The key problem of psychiatric anthropology. In J. Casagrande and T. Gladwin, (Eds.), *Some uses of anthropology, theoretical and applied*, pp. 23-48. Washington, D.C.

Drabkin, I.E. (1974). Remarks on ancient psychopathology. In K.J. Dover, (Ed.), *Greek Popular morality in the time of Plato and Aristotle.* Berkeley: University of California Press.

Dube, K.C. (1985). Psychiatric training and therapies in Ayurveda. *American Journal of Chinese Medicine, 13*, 13-22.

Dube, K.C. (1978). Nosology and therapy of mental illness in Ayurveda. *Comparative Medicine East and West, 6*(3), 209-228.

Edgerton, R. (1969). On the "recognition" of mental illness. In R. Edgerton and S.C. Ploy, (Eds.), *Changing perspectives in mental illness, pp. 49-72.* New York: Holt, Rinehart and Winston.

Fabrega, H., Jr. (1974). *Disease and social behavior: An interdisciplinary perspective.* Cambridge, Massachusetts: Massachusetts Institute and Technology Press.

Fabrega, H., Jr. (1975). The position of psychiatry in the understanding of human disease. *Archives of General Psychiatry. 32*, 1500-1512.

Fabrega, H., Jr. (1976). The function of medical systems. *Perspectives of Biology and Medicine, 20*(1), 108-112.

Fabrega, H., Jr. (1980). The position of psychiatric illness in biomedical theory: A cultural analysis. *Journal of Medicine and Philosophy, 5*(2), 145-168.

Fabrega, H., Jr. (1989a). On the significance of an anthropological approach to schizophrenia. *Psychiatry, 52*, 45-64.

Fabrega, H., Jr. (1989b). The self and schizophrenia: A cultural perspective. *Schizophrenia Bulletin, 15*(2), 277-290.

Fabrega, H., Jr. (1989c). Cultural relativism and psychiatric illness. *Journal of Nervous and Mental Disease, 177*(7), 415-425.

Fabrega, H., Jr. (1989d). An ethnomedical perspective of Anglo-American psychiatry. *American Journal of Psychiatry, 146*(5), 588-596.

Geuss, R. (1981). *The idea of a critical theory.* Cambridge: Cambridge University Press.

Gwei-Djewn, L. & Needham, J. (1980). *Celestial lancets: A history and rationale of acupuncture and moxa.* Cambridge: Cambridge University Press.

Haldipur, C.V. (1984). Madness in ancient India: Concept of insanity in Charaka Samhita (1st Century A.D.). *Comprehensive Psychiatry, 25*(3), 335-344.

Hoenig, J. (1983). The concept of schizophrenia: Kraepelin-Bleuler-Schneider. *British Journal of Psychiatry*, *142*, 547-556.

Hoenig, J. (1982). Kurt Schneider and Anglophone psychiatry. *Comprehensive Psychiatry*, *23*(5), 391-400.

Hollis, M. & Lukes, S. (Eds). (1982). *Rationality and relativism*. Cambridge: Massachusetts Institute and Technology Press.

Hudson R.P. (1983). *Disease and its control: The shaping of modern thought*. Connecticut: Greenwood Press.

Jackson S.W. (1969). Galen - on mental disorders. *Journal of the History of Behavioral Science*, *5*, 365-384.

Jackson S.W. (1970). Force and kindred notions in eighteenth-century neurophysiology and medical psychology. *Bulletin of the History of Medicine*, *44*, 397-554.

Jackson, S.W. (1972). Unusual Mental States in Medieval Europe. I Medical Syndromes of Mental Disorders: 400-1100 A.D. *Journal of the History of Medicine and Allied Sciences*, *27*, 262-297.

Jeste, D.V., et al. (1985). Did schizophrenia exist before the eighteenth century? *Comprehensive Psychiatry*, *26*(6), 493-503.

Kety, S. (1980). The syndrome of schizophrenia: unresolved questions and opportunities for research. *British Journal of Psychiatry*, *136*, 421-436.

Kinnier Wilson, J.V. (1967). *Mental diseases of ancient Mesopotamia*. In D. Brothwell and A.T. Sandison, (Eds.), *Diseases in antiquity*. Illinois: CC Thomas.

Kleinman, A.M. (1975). The symbolic context of Chinese medicine: A comparative approach to the study of traditional medical and psychiatric forms of care in Chinese culture. *American Journal of Chinese Medicine*, *3*(2), 103-124.

Kleinman, A. (1988). *Rethinking psychiatry: From cultural category to personal experience*. New York: Macmillan, Free Press.

Kutumbiah, P. (1969). *Ancient Indian medicine*. Revised Edition. Bombay: Orient Longman.

Leslie, C. (1976). *Asian medical systems*. Berkeley: University of California Press.

Lin, K.M. (1981). Traditional Chinese medicine beliefs and their relevance for mental illness and psychiatry. In A. Kleinman and T.Y. Lin, (Eds.), *Normal and abnormal behavior in Chinese culture*, pp. 95-114. Reidel: Dordrecht.

Lopez-Pinero, J.M. (1983). *Historical origins of the concept of neurosis*. Cambridge: Cambridge University Press.

Moss, G.C. (1967). Mental disorder in antiquity. In D. Brothwell and A.T. Sandison, (Eds.), *Diseases in antiquity*, pp. 709-722. Illinois: CC Thomas.

Murphy, J.M. (1976). Psychiatric labeling in cross-cultural perspective. *Science*, *191*, 1019-28.

Neuburger, M. (1945). British and German psychiatry in the second half of the eighteenth and the early nineteenth century. *Bulletin of the History of Medicine*, *18*, 121-145.

Neugebauer, R. (1976). *Mental illness and government policy in sixteenth and seventeenth century England*. (Ph.D. Thesis). New York: Columbia University.

Neugebauer, R. (1979). Medieval and early modern theories of mental illness. *Archives of General Psychiatry*, *36*, 477.

Nutton, V. (1983). The seeds of disease: An explanation of contagion and infection from the Greeks to the renaissance. *Medicine in History*, *27*, 1-34.

Nutton, V. (1984). From Galen to Alexander: Aspects of medicine and medical practice in late antiquity. In J. Scarborough (Ed.), *Symposium on Byzantine medicine*, No. 38, pp. 1-14. Washington, DC: Dumbarton Oaks Paper.

Nutton, V. (1985). Murders and miracles: Lay attitudes towards medicine in antiquity. In R. Porter (Ed.), *Patients and practitioners: Lay perceptions of medicine in Pre-industrial society*, pp. 25-53. Cambridge: Cambridge University Press.

Obeyesekere, G. (1977). The theory and practice of Ayurvedic medicine in the Ayurvedic tradition. *Culture, Medicine and Psychiatry*, *1*, 155-181.

Pagel, W. (1972). Van Helmont's concept of disease - to be or not to be? The influence of Paracelsus. *Bulletin of the History of Medicine, 46*, 419-454.

Pagel, W. & Winder, M. (1968). Harvey and the "modern" concept of disease. *Bulletin of the History of Medicine, 42*, 496-509.

Parsons, T. (1951). *The social system*. New York: Free Press.

Rao, A.V. (1975). India. In J.G. Howells, (Ed.), *World history of psychiatry*. New York: Brunner/Mazel.

Rather, L.J. (1959). Towards a philosophical study of the idea of disease. In C. McBrooks and P.F. Cranefield (Eds.), *The historical development of physiological thought*. pp. 351-373. New York: Hafner.

Riese, W. (1945). History and principles of classification of nervous diseases. *Bulletin of the History of Medicine, 18*, 465-512.

Riese, W. (1960). The impact of 19th century thought on psychiatry. *International Record of Medicine, 173*, 7-19.

Rosen, G. (1968). *Madness in society*. Chicago: University of Chicago Press.

Saunders, J.B. de C.M. (1963). *The transitions from ancient Egyptian to Greek medicine*, pp. 1-40. Lawrence: University of Kansas Press.

Scharfetter, C. (1975). The historical development of the concept of schizophrenia. In M.H. Laded (Ed.), *Studies of schizophrenia*. London: Headley Brothers.

Schepper-Hughes, N. & Lock, N. (1986). Speaking truth to illness: Metaphors, reifications and a pedagogy for patients. *Medical Anthropology Quarterly, 17*, 137-140.

Schiffeler, J.W. (1979). An essay on some of the fundamental philosophical tenets found in traditional Chinese medicine. *American Journal of Chinese Medicine, 7*(3), 285-294.

Scull, A. (1979). *Museums of madness*. New York: St. Martin's Press.

Shweder R.A. (1990). Cultural psychology: What is it? In J.W. Stigler, R.A. Shweder and G. Herdt (Eds.), *Cultural psychology: The Chicago symposia on culture and human development*, pp. 1-43. New York: Cambridge University Press.

Silverman, J. (1967). Shamans and acute Schizophrenia. *American Anthropologist, 69*, 21-31.

Simon, B. (1978). *Mind and madness in ancient Greece*. New York: Cornell University Press.

Simons, R.C. & Hughes, C.C. (1985). *The culture-bound syndromes*. Boston: Reidel.

Spiro, M.E. (1986). Cultural relativism and the future of anthropology. *Cultural Anthropology, 1*(3), 259-286.

Temkin, O. (1963). The scientific approach to disease: specific entity and individual sickness. In A.C. Clembie (Ed.), *Scientific change*, pp. 629-647. New York: Basic Books.

Temkin, O. (1971). *The falling sickness - A history of epilepsy from the Greeks to the beginnings of modern neurology*. Baltimore: The Johns Hopkins Press.

Tseng, W.S. (1973). The development of psychiatric concepts in traditional Chinese medicine. *Archives of General Psychiatry, 29*, 569-575.

Unschuld, P.U. (1983). *Medicine in China: A history of pharmaceutics*. Berkeley: University of California Press.

Weiss, M. (1977). *Critical study of Unmada in the early Sanskrit medical literature*. (Ph.D. Dissertation), University of Pennsylvania.

Wilson, B.R. (Ed.) (1970). *Rationality*. London: Blackwell.

Yanchi, L. (1988a). *The essential book of traditional Chinese medicine*, Volume I: Theory. New York: Columbia University Press.

Yanchi, L. (1988b). *The essential book of traditional Chinese medicine*, Volume II: Clinical practice. New York: Columbia University Press.

11
Defining Schizophrenia: A Critique of the Mechanistic Framework

Daniel R. Miller
William F. Flack, Jr.

The Problem of Definition

On initial consideration, defining schizophrenia does not seem to be a pressing problem for the clinician or researcher. Among the various professionals whose work impinges on the lives of psychotic patients, there is a working consensus concerning the definition developed and codified in the *Diagnostic and Statistical Manual* (DSM-III-R) of the American Psychiatric Association (1987). Beneath the surface of apparent agreement, however, there is evidence of considerable disagreement. Even apart from the carpings of academicians and philosophers whose function it is to cast doubt on seemingly clear conceptions, the writings of both theorists and clinicians reveal radical differences in their pictures of the disorder. Many examples of these differences may be found in a group of articles written in answer to the question "What is schizophrenia?" The responses, which were published in the *Schizophrenia Bulletin* between 1982 to 1984, reveal a mixed bag of conceptions and much disagreement about criteria, underlying assumptions, and even the nature and purposes of definitions.

The pressure for a clear and workable conception is created by the fact that psychiatrists, psychologists, social workers, nurses, judges, and administrators must make daily decisions about diagnosis and treatment. To have confidence in their decisions, these professionals must have confidence in their conceptions of schizophrenia and be able to differentiate it from syndromes with similar symptoms. Obtaining such confidence is unfortunately a daunting goal. For almost one hundred years, investigators have been studying schizophrenia by means of an impressive variety of techniques. Much empirical knowledge has been amassed, but the research has not yet yielded a theoretical basis for obtaining a consensus about criteria. In the absence of a consensus, it is not surprising that many definitions have been proposed, and that the American Psychiatric Association, the arbiter of definitions, keeps changing its criteria.

At the present time, a perusal of the literature on the meaning of schizophrenia is like a stroll through a street market in which various hawkers of what are proclaimed to be similar wares appeal to the consumer in their own idiosyncratic languages. The range of definitions is by no means exhausted by the following examples: a disorder of dopamine metabolism (Carlton & Manowitz, 1984); an affective disturbance (Bleuler, 1911/1950); a genetic disposition (Gottesman, 1990); a form of deteriorated functioning (Kraepelin, 1919); a disturbance in familial interaction (Dell, 1980); a spoiling of identity (Sarbin & Mancuso, 1980); a learning of inappropriate responses (Ullman & Krasner, 1975); a regression caused by internal conflict (Klein, 1946); a relationship involving a pseudocommunity and social exclusion (Lemert, 1951); a disturbance in the ability to communicate (Bateson, Jackson, Haley, & Weakland, 1956); and a fortuitous labeling of people who are then socialized in the role of the mad patient (Scheff, 1966).

The variety of notions inevitably raises doubts about whether different investigators are studying the same phenomenon. Since there are no external criteria, it is not possible for the working clinician to reconcile the differences among different versions of schizophrenia, or to make rational choices from among them. Faced with the necessity of making daily decisions crucial to their patients' welfare, clinicians tend to cling unquestioningly to the criteria of the Diagnostic and Statistical Manual, fearful of questioning their veridicality in view of the lack of alternatives sanctioned by respected authorities. Unclear about ways to formulate criteria on a theoretical basis, some writers think these efforts are a waste of time and that investigators would do better to concentrate on further empirical investigations.

Sources of Disagreement

A review of the different conceptions of schizophrenia reveals more disagreement than agreement on most fundamental issues. Some writers do not even acknowledge that there is such a pathological condition, whether or not it is called schizophrenia. Those who postulate such a condition are not in agreement about whether it is one or a number of different states, whether there is a universal group of symptoms or if the syndrome varies with the society, whether the disorder is learned or genetically determined, or whether it is a disturbance in the functioning of the society, the family, the social relationship, or the individual.

There are at least three major reasons for this conceptual Tower of Babel. One is the diversity in frames of reference. Classifications may differ, for example, with respect to their purposes. The system devised to help the practicing clinician may differ from the one devised by the administrator, who is more interested in allocating patients to open or closed wards, and in categorizing them for purposes of making insurance claims. Systems also tend to vary with the authors' professional training, which inevitably creates predilections for thinking in genetic, biochemical, psychological, or sociological terms. Implicit in these professionally determined orientations are premises and questions that make it difficult to relate the research of investigators from different professions. One is often hard put, for example, to formulate connections between findings about the learning of particular responses, their genetic transmission, and their apparent transformations in latah, village idiocy, and other pathologies in different societies.

In this chapter we focus primarily on two other sources of diversity. One pertains to differences about the significance of theory for the derivation of criteria. Some writers begin with specific theoretical premises, while others, like the authors of the Diagnostic and Statistical Manual, eschew theory in favor of subjective assessment and blindly empirical methods. The second source of diversity is created by differences in philosophical positions.

The philosophical biases of the authors of the standard version of schizophrenia lead them to think of it as both a mental condition and a physical disease akin to many of those for which cures have been developed by medical researchers. They also think that medicine is a value-free science akin to physics. Hence, they try to formulate principles that have been reduced as closely as possible to the elements of mechanics; principles that can be defined objectively and that have the same meaning in every society. In contrast, there are other writers who view pathology as a problem for societal stability, and who think it is not fruitful to use the reductionistic concepts of mechanics. Much of the remainder of this chapter is devoted to these disagreements about methodology and philosophical assumptions.

Dementia Praecox and Schizophrenia

The definition of schizophrenia in DSM-III-R is the latest in a series of revisions that began with Kraepelin's (1919) proposal of the syndrome of dementia praecox. We begin with a short review of his thinking because we feel it established a viewpoint and a methodology that have been followed to this day.

To derive the syndrome, Kraepelin first identified clinically a particular group of patients and made sure that all of them had the properties that his experience had led him to expect. A longitudinal study had convinced him that this group had two salient properties: the disorder starts early, and it gradually culminates in the deterioration of certain mental functions. Hence the term, "dementia praecox."

Kraepelin's observations of these patients also led him to include in his criteria three pathological characteristics that had previously been regarded as discrete types of disorder—catatonia, hebephrenia, and paranoia. Contrary to previous investigators, he found that these types of disorders occurred in his criterion group. Finally, his clinical studies led him to include the additional symptoms of hallucinations, delusions, emotional blunting, disorders of thought with unusual associations, negativism, and decrease in attention toward the outer world.

In the second part of his method, Kraepelin compared his patients who had dementia praecox with groups who had other pathologies, and selected as identifying properties only those that were not characteristic of the patients with other disorders. The purpose of this step was to insure that there was minimal overlap between the attributes of patients identified as having dementia praecox and those of the other groups.

However, a similar quest for symptoms that exist only in the group under study led Bleuler (1911/1950) to propose radical changes in Kraepelin's syndrome. Bleuler's clinical impressions prompted him to reject Kraepelin's criteria of dementia and early onset, and to relinquish the method of temporal analysis by which they were derived. Instead, he proposed that the syndrome be divided into primary and secondary categories. Primary symptoms are always present, and attributable to a presumed etiological agent. The secondary symptoms are products of psychological reactions to the primary ones. They are not always present, but they affect the clinical picture when they are.

In proposing a new name, schizophrenia, which referred to a personality split by unusual combinations of associations, Bleuler made Kraepelin's criterion of thought disorder the foremost of the primary symptoms, which also included disturbances of affectivity, a predilection for fantasy as opposed to reality, and an inclination to divorce oneself from reality. Hallucinations, delusions, and catatonia were demoted to the secondary category of reactive symptoms, which also included various behavioral disturbances.

The Current Definition

Official definitions of schizophrenia have been revised a number of times. The authors of the current American version, which is strongly influenced by the writings of Schneider (1959), emphasize that they do not justify it on theoretical grounds. They continue to use Kraepelin's method of seeking maximal differentiation between different groups identified on the basis of clinical impression.

The syndrome described in DSM-III-R includes various types of delusions and hallucinations, loosening of associations, catatonic behavior, inappropriate affect, deterioration of social comportment, and a group of social malfunctions that are either prodromal or residual. The authors justify some of these changes solely because they are consistent with Kraepelin's thinking (Kendler, Spitzer, & Williams, 1989). Certainly, their conception of schizophrenia is a far cry from Bleuler's. It discards or diminishes the significance of his primary symptoms, and eliminates his distinction between them and symptoms in the secondary category. Its diagnostic criteria include two members of Bleuler's secondary group, symptoms he considers "unessential in that they appear or disappear without altering the essence of the disease" (1911/1950). Finally, the DSM-III-R restores temporal criteria. So different is the current version of schizophrenia from Bleuler's version that Kety (1985) protests, with justification, that the authors should have coined another name in order to avoid confusion with the term schizophrenia. Reliance on the experience of clinical authority provides a shaky foundation, then, for the development of criteria for identifying patients with a particular syndrome, particularly when the authorities disagree, and classifiers of different generations differ on the authority to whom they decide to pay homage.

Evaluative Criteria

Although Bleuler had no theoretical basis for constructing his syndrome, he suggests some valuable criteria for judging whether a particular construction refers to a discriminable and cohesive entity. First, he proposed that the term must include symptoms that occur only and always in the clinically identified group. In other words, they do not overlap with the symptoms of any other entity. Second, no one set of symptoms can be singled out that does not show definite connections with all the others; they are significantly interrelated. Finally, the concept corresponds to reality in that the criteria can be discovered very easily. Fortunately, there are sufficient empirical data to permit a judgment of the adequacy of the definition of schizophrenia in the light of Bleuler's criteria.

Despite Bleuler's stated confidence in his concept, he qualifies the use of his criteria. For example, he states that the symptoms must have reached a certain degree of intensity to be of diagnostic value. Even in the most advanced cases, however, the symptoms are not necessarily present all the time; several hours of assessment may not be sufficient to establish the diagnosis. Moreover, some are so subtle that their identification can be made only in terms of the circumstances in which they occur. He also acknowledges that there are mild and latent forms of the disease that are very difficult to diagnose. Finally, he assumes that schizophrenic symptoms are distortions and exaggerations of normal processes. Hence, he is open to the possibility that non-schizophrenics may develop symptoms such as auditory hallucinations, and that some schizophrenics may have states of clear consciousness. In short, he concedes at the outset that the syndrome overlaps to some extent with non-schizophrenic ones.

1. The Criterion of Minimal Overlap

The amount of possible overlap is much greater in the current version of schizophrenia as described in DSM-III-R. To begin with, there is a Residual Type, which lacks the essential symptoms of delusions, hallucinations, incoherence, and behavior disorganization, but is still regarded as schizophrenia. But some residual symptoms (marked lack of initiative, marked impairment in role functioning as wage earner, student, or homemaker, blunted or inappropriate affect) are likely to overlap with those of a number of non-schizophrenic disorders.

Overlap is magnified further by the inclusion in the Diagnostic and Statistical Manual of a group of disorders that, although they are classified as being different from schizophrenia, have some of its characteristics. For example, Delusional (Paranoid) Disorder is identified by delusions that are "nonbizarre" and hallucinations that are not prominent; Brief Reactive Psychosis conforms to all the criteria for schizophrenia except for prodromal symptoms and duration; Schizophreniform Disorder fails to meet the criteria for disorganized social behavior and duration; Schizoaffective Disorder combines manic or depressive symptoms with schizophrenic ones; Mood Disorders with Psychotic Features includes delusions, hallucinations, or catatonic symptoms; Schizoid Personality Disorder contains the social disorganization common in schizophrenia; and Schizotypal Personality Disorder seems to be a milder version of schizophrenia. One wonders just how much agreement there is among even experienced clinicians in their discrimination among these syndromes, not to mention discrimination between each of them and cases of schizophrenia.

Further violations of the criterion of minimal overlap are contained in empirical data that reveal schizophrenic symptoms in patients diagnosed as having functional disorders that would not be expected to overlap with schizophrenia. Delusions are common among patients with affective disorders (Winters & Neale, 1983); hallucinations are frequent in a number of different disorders as well as in normals (Asaad & Shapiro, 1986), (which is probably one reason why Bleuler classified them as secondary symptoms); and thought disorders may be found in patients diagnosed as manic (Andreasen, 1979), depressive, or aphasic (Persons, 1986). Even many normals report psychotic-like experiences (Bentall & Slade, 1985).

2. Other Criteria

Bleuler's second criterion, that the symptoms are significantly associated with one another, is not supported by empirical findings. Factor analysis and cluster analysis produce contradictory results (Blashfield, 1984; Everitt, Gourlay & Kendall, 1971; Slade & Cooper, 1979), but relationships between diagnosis and obtained clusters are weak, at best.

Bleuler's third criterion, that the syndrome corresponds to reality, can be interpreted in different ways, but none seem inconsistent with the requirement of minimal reliability. By this standard, the construct of schizophrenia fares better than it does when judged by the first two criteria. The inter-rater reliability improved significantly following the introduction of operational criteria in the latest version of the Diagnostic and Statistical Manual. But this reliability is based on simultaneous ratings. Reliability based on ratings made at different times is not expected to be high because schizophrenic symptoms appear and disappear unpredictably (Cromwell, 1984).

Researchers have also been judging schizophrenia in terms of a further criterion. If it is assumed that the term refers to a distinct group of disorders, then one would expect the course of the disease and its responses to treatment to differ from those associated with other syndromes. This expectation is not supported by the results. So much variability occurs in the course of the disorder that one investigator (Ciompi, 1980; 1984) rejects the notion of a unitary disease. Strauss & Carpenter (1974; 1977) report considerable overlap in outcome between schizophrenic patients and hospitalized patients with other diagnoses. Moreover, the considerable variability in outcomes is not related to particular symptoms or certainty of diagnosis. Compared to the results for symptoms manifested on admission, performance at work, frequency of social contacts and other social attributes are more strongly related to outcomes.

3. Contradictory Evaluations of Results

These empirical findings have prompted numerous investigators to express serious doubts about the concept valiation of schizophrenia. Typical is the less than lukewarm claim that it is a reification with minimal utility (Cromwell, 1984), and the vote for discarding a construct that "seems to have no particular symptoms, which follows no particular course, and which responds to no (or perhaps every) particular treatment" (Bentall, Jackson, & Pilgrim, 1988, p. 314).

Paradoxically, despite the convincingly negative findings, many clinicians are loathe to reject a concept that they employ daily in diagnosing patients, interpreting symptoms, and conducting therapy. Their commitment to the concept is also bolstered by two articles of faith. One is confidence in the authority of Kraepelin and Bleuler, who proclaimed that schizophrenia exists and is a mental disease. The other is a confidence, engendered by revolutionary medical discoveries in the 19th and 20th centuries, that medical researchers will ultimately discover the etiology of schizophrenia, and devise an effective biochemical treatment.

The Mechanistic Viewpoint In Medicine

It is our impression that many of the fundamental problems inherent in the concept of schizophrenia can be traced to a traditional medical viewpoint that guided the thinking of Kraepelin and Bleuler. It is a viewpoint that is inherent in current attempts to identify and define pathological states. Kraepelin and Bleuler unhesitatingly proclaimed that schizophrenia is a disease. In this section, we examine conceptions of disease as products of three traditions that were integrated during the nineteenth century: a particular scientific doctrine, a mechanical conception of causality, and a reliance on clinical authority.

The dominant medical conception of disease originated in connection with the development of physical medicine in the last century. At that time, medicine was typically viewed as a natural science. This viewpoint was helped by the acceptance of Descartes' duality of mind and body; once mind could be assigned to other disciplines, physicians could devote themselves exclusively to the understanding and curing of bodily ills. Medical education was concentrated on biology, chemistry, and physics. Thus, most physicians were taught to phrase their concepts in the language of the natural sciences and to formulate their problems in mechanistic and deterministic terms.

The mechanistic view provided a frame of reference for many of the most revolutionary discoveries of the nineteenth and twentieth centuries. According to the doctrine of the period, each disease is a unique natural phenomenon identified by its unique pattern of signs and symptoms. Its understanding requires the identification of an agent that is usually external. By various means, it invades the body and inflicts the damage that helps one identify the syndrome. The agent is experienced as something you catch or eat, or which happens to you.

The conception of a disease was formulated in terms of a configuration consisting of signs, symptoms, and physiological laws invoked in terms of the nature of the agent. This configuration was typically reified as an entity. The presumptions that each disease alters specific organs, and that it requires a particular therapy, were probably derived from this doctrine about specific etiology (DuBos, 1959).

1. Philosophical Assumptions

Inherent in the viewpoint of the medical mechanists are three philosophical positions—reductionism, universalism, and objectivity. It is not meaningful to regard such positions as either right or wrong. Being matters of faith, they are significant because they have fundamental impacts on the formation of concepts, the phrasing of questions, and the choice of methods favored by investigators (Miller & Jaques, 1988).

Mechanists are committed reductionists. They feel that the explanation of social phenomena and of psychological states requires their reanalysis first into the concepts of biology, and then, if possible, into the concepts of chemistry and physics. Social and psychological findings are consequently downgraded in favor of physiological and biochemical data. For example, one eminent investigator asserts that "there is no such thing as a psychiatry that is too biological ..." (Hunt, 1990, p. 3). Correspondingly there is widespread doubt among physicians, according to one medical educator (Eisenberg, 1988), that psychological and social factors are as "real" as biological ones: "... physicians continue to be skeptics about social research when they are not downright arrogant in their dismissal of it."

The second position, universalism, follows from the bias in favor of reductionism, according to which medical scientists assume that, to be meaningful, the symptoms of any disease must be reduced to physiological concepts. Hence they must be universal: they must have the same meaning in every society and historical period. Nosologies are useful to the extent that they approximate a "sovereign order of nature" (Pichot, 1986)—one that is presumably independent of culture and history.

Objectivity, the mechanists' third position, is consistent with the first two. A number of theorists have tried to define disease in terms that are compatible with objective biological theory. For Boorse (1977), disease is an impairment of functional ability, a deviation from what is statistically normal for the species design relative to age and sex. His concern with objectivity leads him to restrict his realm of discourse to physiological functions. He defines these as the causal contributions that physical traits or processes make to particular goals, such as other processes of the organism. Goals are organized in a hierarchy, the apex of which is characterized by such examples as individual survival and reproduction. Judgments about functions are value-free, he claims, since estimates of contributions to biological goals are based on empirical findings.

2. The Mechanists' Orientation To Schizophrenia

In support of reductionistic analysis, Bleuler agrees with Kraepelin that disease affects the body, not the mind. He also takes it for granted that a specific etiological agent will ultimately be identified, and that it will affect the structure or functioning of the central nervous system. After describing the clinical manifestations of schizophrenia, Bleuler states that complete justice to the diversity of symptoms can be achieved only by the assumption of a disease that entails the presence of anatomical or chemical disturbances of the brain. These disturbances in turn "determine" the primary symptoms.

The universality of the presumed anatomical or chemical etiology is emphasized by the claim that the incidence of the disease varies neither among the sub-groups of Bleuler's society nor among different societies. Occurence of the disease, he claims, is as frequent among "primitive" peoples as it is among the technologically advanced. He thinks that there are probably no psychic causes of schizophrenia.

To demonstrate that schizophrenia is consistent with the sovereign order of nature, Bleuler devotes considerable effort to showing that the syndrome refers to an "entity." The syndrome actually exists, he claims, and its characteristics are discernable by objective observation.

3. Problems Created by the Mechanistic Framework

Given their reductionist views, Kraepelin and Bleuler would have preferred to employ biochemical and anatomical methods of diagnosis. But at the time, too little was known about brain pathology and techniques for studying it. Information about the presumed disease could be gleaned only from psychic events. Thus, despite their principles, Kraepelin and Bleuler were forced to utilize psychological data in their explorations of the nature of schizophrenia.

This mechanistic orientation has created a number of problems for modern psychiatrists, whose options have tended to be restricted by many of the conceptions and procedures used in 1911. Although many new techniques have become available, methods of diagnosis have tended to be restricted to the clinical interview. Strong faith in reductionism has helped to generate a large amount of productive biochemical and genetic research. However, it has encouraged tendencies to formulate problems in terms of atomistic variables, and to neglect the molar concepts that are most frequently used in psychological, sociological, and anthropological research. It has also led the majority of clinicians to neglect the vast literature on the cross-cultural expression of psychosis.

Most serious are the problems stemming from dependence on clinical authority. One problem is the reluctance on the part of committees who devise conceptions of schizophrenia to be explicit about the theoretical assumptions that are obviously inherent in present methods of classification. Another is the inclination to ignore research that is relevant to the formulation of diagnostic criteria.

The unwillingness to theorize has created a serious barrier to the improvement of diagnostic criteria. As Kaplan (1964) observes, even apparently simple spatio-temporal identifications entail heavy commitments to implicit theories. Conceptualization, he observes, informs the perceptual process from the beginning. Kaplan adds that it is unrealistic to place much faith on strict or original definitions before the necessary empirical information is available. Unless concepts are formulated on the basis of sound empirical work, important areas of investigation may be dismissed prematurely.

Possible Bases for Change

It might be fruitful for new versions of the DSM if their authors took into account a number of findings for which there is abundant clinical evidence. There is considerable evidence (Strauss, this volume) of sequential changes in the patterns of symptoms displayed by the same person; a patient may be depressed for a while, shift to schizophrenia, and then revert to depression. Because of a commitment to a structural view of disease as a static entity, changeless in time, clinicians ignore this evidence and make a diagnosis by watching the patient for a time and making a primary diagnosis, presuming that this is the underlying changeless one.

Also relevant to systems of classification is evidence that the phasic manifestations of symptoms require repeated testing if the clinician is to have any confidence in the validity of the diagnosis (Carson & Sanislow, in press; Cromwell, 1984); the confounding effects on diagnosis of symptoms resulting from treatment and institutionalization (Wing & Brown, 1970); the greater predictive validity of the negative symptoms than the positive ones which monopolize the criteria of DSM-III (negative symptoms referring to the absence of expected attributes such as self-support and maintenance of social relationships) (Strauss & Carpenter, 1981); the pertinence of current criteria of schizophrenia primarily to a relatively late stage of the disorder (Strauss & Carpenter, 1981); support for Kraepelin's currently deemphasized temporal analysis; and support for the currently discarded differentiation, originally proposed by Bleuler, between primary and secondary symptoms.

Future authors of the DSM would also do well to review some of the cogent criticisms of philosophical positions implicit in current methods of nosological formulation. Most relevant are the publications of Brown (1985), Carson (1984), Dubos (1965), Engelhardt (1975), Feinstein (1976), Miller & Jaques (1988), and Whitbeck (1978). Finally, some specialists might break out of the confines of their mechanistic frame of reference if they considered other medical and non-medical models.

Particularly challenging to the mechanistic viewpoint is the work of Dubos (1959; 1965), who criticizes the espousal of reductionism and objectivity, replaces the idea of a simple etiological agent with a system of complex causality, proposes that systems of classification are products of the society's collective judgment, and illustrates the relevance to classification of environmental conditions, social norms and values, the history of the group, and the individual's aspirations. Some examples of non-medical models are Parsons' (1951) analysis of medical classification as a means of societal control, Miller & Jaques' (1988) view of psychosis as dysfunctional attributes that interfere with coordination of socially required activities, Rosenberg's (1984) interpretation of schizophrenia as a problem in taking the role of the other, and Goffman's (1983) conception of infelicitous social behavior as a disturbance in metacommunication.

It seems probable that comparisons of such different systems might help to disentangle some of the confusions about methodological and philosophical issues underlying the thinking about classifying pathologies. There are many such issues, a fact that explains the formidable problems faced by the classifiers. But there is basis for optimism that the identification of these issues will lay a groundwork that may clarify their importance to the definition of pathologies like schizophrenia.

References

American Psychiatric Association (1987). *Diagnostic and statistical manual of mental disorders, 3rd edition, revised.* Washington, DC: Author.

Andreasen, N.C. (1979). Thought, language and communication disorders: II. Diagnostic significance. *Archives of General Psychiatry, 36*, 1325-1330.

Asaad, G. & Shapiro, M.D. (1986). Hallucinations: Theoretical and clinical overview. *American Journal of Psychiatry, 143*, 1088-1097.

Bateson, G., Jackson, D.D., Haley, J., & Weakland, J.H. (1956). Toward a theory of schizophrenia. *Behavioral Science, 1*, 251-264.

Blashfield, R.K. (1984). *The classification of psychopathology: Neo-Kraepelinian and quantitative approaches.* New York: Plenum.

Bentall, R.P., Jackson, H.F., & Pilgrim, D. (1988). Abandoning the concept of 'schizophrenia:' Some implications of validity arguments for psychological research into psychotic phenomena. *British Journal of Clinical Psychology, 27*, 303-324.

Bentall, R.P. & Slade, P.D. (1985). Reliability of a scale designed to measure predisposition to hallucination. *Personality and Individual Differences, 6*, 527-529.

Bleuler, E. (1911/1950). *Dementia praecox or the group of schizophrenias.* NY: International Universities Press.

Boorse, C. (1977). Health as a theoretical concept. *Philosophy of Science, 44*, 542-573.

Brown, W.M. (1985). On defining "disease." *Journal of Medicine and Philosophy, 10*, 311-328.

Carlton, P.L. & Manowitz, P. (1984). Dopamine and schizophrenia: An analysis of the theory. *Neuroscience & Biobehavioral Reviews, 8*, 137-151.

Carson, R.C. (1984). The schizophrenias. In H.E. Adams & P.B. Sutker (Eds.), *Comprehensive handbook of psychopathology.* NY: Plenum.

Carson, R.C. & Sanislow, C.A., III (in press). The schizophrenias. In H.E. Adams & P.B. Sutker (Eds.), *Comprehensive handbook of psychopathology, 2nd edition.* NY: Plenum.

Ciompi, L. (1980). The natural history of schizophrenia in the long term. *British Journal of Psychiatry, 136*, 413-420.

Ciompi, L. (1984). Is there really a schizophrenia? The long-term course of psychotic phenomena. *British Journal of Psychiatry, 145*, 636-640.

Cromwell, R.L. (1984). Preemptive thinking and schizophrenia research. In W.D. Spaulding & J.K. Cole (Eds.), *Theories of schizophrenia and psychosis: Nebraska symposium on motivation,* Volume 31. Lincoln, NE: University of Nebraska Press.

Dell, P.F. (1980). Researching the family theories of schizophrenia: An exercise in epistemological confusion. *Family Process, 19* (4), 321-335.

Dubos, R. (1959). *Mirage of health: Utopias, progress, and biological change.* New Brunswick, NJ: Rutgers University Press.

Dubos, R. (1965). *Man adapting*. New Haven, CT: Yale University Press.

Eisenberg, L. (1988). Science in medicine: Too much, too little and too limited in scope? *American Journal of Medicine, 84*, 483-490.

Engelhardt, H.T., Jr. (1975). The concepts of health and disease. In H.T. Engelhardt & S.F. Spicker (Eds.), *Evaluation and explanation in the biomedical sciences*. Dordrecht-Holland: D. Reidel Publishing Company.

Everitt, B.S., Gourlay, A.J., & Kendell, R.E. (1971). An attempt at validation of traditional psychiatric syndromes by cluster analysis. *British Journal of Psychiatry, 119*, 399-412.

Feinstein, (1976). *Clinical judgment*. Huntington, NY: R.E. Krieger Publishing Company.

Goffman, E. (1983). Felicity's condition. *American Journal of Sociology, 89* (1), 1-53.

Gottesman, I.I. (1990). *Schizophrenia genesis: The origins of madness*. NY: W.H. Freeman and Company.

Hunt, M. (1990). Genetics in psychiatry: An essential tool. *NARSAD Research Newsletter*, 1-2.

Kaplan, A. (1964). *The conduct of inquiry: Methodology for behavioral science*. San Francisco: Chandler Publishing Company.

Kendler, K.S., Spitzer, R.L., & Williams, J.B.W. (1989). Psychotic disorders in DSM-III-R. *American Journal of Psychiatry, 146* (8), 953-962.

Kety, S.S. (1985). The concept of schizophrenia. In M. Alpert (Ed.), *Controversies in schizophrenia: Changes and constancies*. NY: The Guilford Press.

Klein, M. (1946). Notes on some schizoid mechanisms. *International Journal of Psycho-Analysis, 27*, 99-110.

Kraepelin, E. (1919). *Dementia praecox and paraphrenia*. Huntington, NY: Robert E. Krieger Publishing Company.

Lemert, C. (1951). *Social pathology*. New York: McGraw-Hill.

Miller, D.R. & Jaques, E. (1988). Identifying madness: An interaction frame of reference. In H.J. O'Gorman (Ed.), *Surveying social life: Essays in honor of Hubert H. Hyman*. Middletown, CT: Wesleyan University Press.

Parsons, T. (1951). *The Social System*. NY: Free Press.

Persons, J.B. (1986). The advantages of studying psychological phenomena rather than psychiatric diagnoses. *American Psychologist, 41*, 1252-1260.

Pichot, P. (1986). Bases and theories of classification in psychiatry. In G. Friedman, et al. (Eds.), *Issues in psychiatric classification: Science, practice & social policy*. NY: Human Sciences Press.

Rosenberg, M. (1984). A symbolic interactionist view of psychosis. *Journal of Health and Social Behavior, 25* (3), 289-302.

Sarbin, T.R. & Mancuso, J.C. (1980). *Schizophrenia: Medical diagnosis or moral verdict?* Elmsford, NY: Pergamon Press.

Scheff, T.J. (1966). *Being mentally ill: A sociological theory*. NY: Aldine Publishing Company.

Schneider, K. (1959). *Clinical psychopathology*. NY: Grune and Stratton.

Slade, P.D. & Cooper, R. (1979). Some conceptual difficulties with the term 'schizophrenia:' An alternative model. *British Journal of Social and Clinical Psychology, 18*, 309-317.

Strauss, J.S. & Carpenter, W.T., Jr. (1974). Prediction of outcome in schizophrenia. II. Relationships between predictor and outcome variables. *Archives of General Psychiatry, 31*, 37-42.

Strauss, J.S. & Carpenter, W.T., Jr. (1977). Prediction of outcome in schizophrenia. III. Five-year outcome and its predictors. *Archives of General Psychiatry, 34*, 159-163.

Strauss, J.S. & Carpenter, W.T., Jr. (1981). *Schizophrenia*. New York: Plenum Medical Book Company.

Ullmann, L. & Krasner, L. (1975). *A psychological approach to abnormal behavior*, 2nd edition. Englewood Cliffs, NJ: Prentice-Hall.

Wing, J.K. & Brown, G.W. (1970). *Institutionalism and schizophrenia: A comparative study of three mental hospitals 1960-1968*. Cambridge, England: Cambridge University Press.

Winters, K.C. & Neale, J.M. (1983). Delusions and delusional thinking in psychotics: A review of the literature. *Clinical Psychology Review, 3*, 227-253.

12
The Grammar of Schizophrenia
Jeff Coulter

Introduction

An invitation to comment on papers dealing with my first professional and intellectual interest, the schizophrenias, was impossible to resist, even though I have not been closely involved in the field for some time, having attempted over the past ten years or so to develop a broader, sociological and philosophical approach to cognitive and "mental" phenomena beyond those characteristically associated with insanity or mental disorders. This, then, was an opportunity to re-visit familiar territory and to discern to what extent the theoretical traditions within which I had been working (Wittgenstein, ethnomethodology) could enable me to speak to the issues which had originally led me to the view that *every* putatively "mental" property of a human agent (and not just the "pathologically" mental, as earlier versions of "labeling theory" proposed[1]) is culturally—intersubjectively- constituted within a matrix of analyzable social interactions and relations: the self-

---

[1]For a useful compendium of "labeling theory" papers, see Scheff (1975). An important theoretical move away from the quasi-etiological claims and metaphysical emphases of traditional labeling theory, with its apparently "arbitrarian," power-driven view of psychiatric diagnosis, was developed quite early by Blum (1970) in a much neglected paper, influenced by the logical analyses of the later Wittgenstein, that still sustained a constructionist, sociological approach to psychiatric phenomena. Although labeling-theoretic ideas exercised a major influence within interactionist sociology through most of the 1960s and very early 1970s, more rigorous ethnomethodological ideas about the social 'logic' of 'membership categorization' practices in general began to replace these earlier formulations, as evidenced in papers such as Smith (1978). Finally, the work of Pollner (1974; 1978) especially his two related critical treatments of "labeling theory" from an ethnomethodological point of view, effectively reoriented serious sociological work away from many of the presuppositions of the conventional "labeling" perspective (especially its assumption of consensual arbitrariness in relation to "deviant behavior") while still retaining an essentially social-constructionist orientation.

subsisting, autonomous "psyche" or Cartesian "res cogitans" is a fiction. The phenomena generally subsumed under the category of the mental (thinking, understanding, hallucinating, imagining, believing, etc.) are not thereby being *denied* (as in some radical versions of behavioristic theory) but are subject to a de-reifying logical and sociological analysis designed to exhibit the properties they actually have.

"Schizophrenia" remains an excellent topic for analysis in terms of this broader controversy. In various respects this issue is a test case for the capacity of social-constructionist inquiry to contribute meaningfully to our understanding of (several of) the ontological and epistemological problems which it raises.

Psychiatric Classification

Any classification system can be assessed as either useful or useless depending upon the purposes of a user; and, while some *particular* classification may be wrong or incorrect, it makes no sense to suppose that an entire scheme of classification may be so designated. A particular move made by a chess-player may be wrong or incorrect, but the game of chess itself is neither right nor wrong, neither correct nor incorrect. In this sense, then, it is simply not a meaningful question to ask: is the taxonomy of Emil Kraepelin which contains the category "schizophrenia" (and its sub-types) right or wrong, correct or incorrect? Rather, we must ask ourselves: is the categorical system useful or usable for the range of purposes for which it is characteristically used? This takes us immediately to the question: what *are* the typical purposes for which the concepts expressed in the classification system are used, and to what extent do the rules governing the use of these concepts facilitate (or hinder) the pursuit of the objectives of their users?

In posing this question, I shall discuss some of the arguments raised by my co-contributors in this volume, restricting myself to contemporary concerns surrounding the use of the concept of schizophrenia; whatever utility such a category may or may not have had for various *historical* purposes, my only consideration here is to assess some of its contemporary uses, purposes of use, and consequences of use. As a first step, then, we must distinguish between two very general kinds of contexts and purposes within which, and for which, the concept/category "schizophrenia" is used: the *clinical-psychiatric* (practical, if you will) and the *research-psychopathological* (theoretical) domains. My impression of some of the discussions that took place at the symposium is that these two related but independently specifiable enterprises were too often conflated, with the result that those who cast doubt upon the instrumental utility of the concept for etiological research purposes were thought thereby to be questioning the pragmatic utility of the concept for treatment-related diagnostic purposes.

I want to argue that while there can be little doubt, as Professor Kendell observes, that the category of "schizophrenia" has proven itself to be useful to psychiatrists for three quarters of a century and that clinical psychiatrists are unlikely to be moved to abandon it on abstract, epistemological grounds, there remain vexed questions about its utility in facilitating the production of uniform, standardized, or replicable samples of instances or "cases" for rigorous scientific inquiry. Many behavioral-science researchers have presented very compelling proposals in professional and technical quarters for the abandonment of the Bleuler-Kraepelin diagnostic categories for research purposes, especially "schizophrenia,"[2] on a variety of grounds. When defined as a Sydenham-type "syndrome," clinical descriptions of its characteristics and reliability of its diagnosis for the purpose of generating comparable, homogeneous samples of cases have been generally unsatisfactory. Even if we grant the wisdom of Professor Zubin's warning against demanding too much rigor in this domain "lest we bring on rigor mortis," it may very well be the case that failures to produce consistent operationalizations and comparable criteria across the landscape of schizophrenia research are functions of the attempt to regiment this core concept's usage beyond its latitudes of tolerance. You cannot, after all, make the concept of a "heap" more exact by piling on operational criteria: it is never going to be amenable to specification by a finitely specifiable set of necessary-and-sufficient conditions as may the concept of a "triangle." Nonetheless, there is no need to throw the baby out with the bathwater; there are plenty of heaps of things in the world, for all our "failures" precisely to pre-specify what constitutes a phenomenon as a "heap," and notwithstanding the uselessness of such a category for measurement purposes in experiments in chemistry or physics. The point, again, is to recollect the diverse purposes for which we deploy our concepts: no science can traffic in "heaps" as it can in "molecules," and perhaps no theoretical psychopathology should be expected to traffic in "schizophrenia" as it can in "epilepsy." However, Professor Kendell and Professor McHugh make strong and eloquent arguments for the possibly continued utility of the category of

---

[2]See, *inter alia*, Angst, 1988; Bentall, 1986; Bentall, et al., 1988; Carpenter & Kirkpatrick, 1988; Ciompi, 1984; Cromwell, 1984; Stephens, et al., 1982.

schizophrenia as a heuristic notion, claiming that reasoning from an assumption of disease in cases where the disease "entity" is, at best, unclear, and even contestable, has sometimes borne fruit, even if the original, research-initiating category is eventually jettisoned at the end of the day (as in the cases of phthisis, which became pulmonary tuberculosis, and myxoedema, which became hypothyroidism). We already have a precedent in the successful extrapolation of Gjessing's syndrome (with its etiological basis known to be a deficit of nitrogen metabolism) from the previously heterodox "catatonias" closer to our immediate interest in the schizophrenic syndrome.

Almost everyone will admit that the categories of schizophrenia resist specification in terms of strict recognition criteria[3] and subsume variably identifiable forms of conduct; differences arise over the conclusions to be derived from this assertion. One line of argument is to propose to substitute particular "symptoms" (e.g., "auditory hallucination") as *explananda* in research programs geared to determining etiological factors, leaving aside the broader issue of the ethical or "sociopolitical" justification for the use of the category in practical psychiatric screening, diagnosis, and treatment. A contrary view is that the persistent troubles encountered in confirming a biological or biochemical justification for the "disease" language of "symptomatology" in relation to the "schizophrenias" should lead us to abandon the disease model as a whole for this domain of inquiry. Professor Sarbin's characterization of this position leads him to argue that what he terms "the schizophrenia hypothesis" (which I shall treat here as meaning the hypothesis that people so diagnosed are suffering from a determinable biological or biochemical abnormality which causes their condition) has already been disconfirmed. The difficulty in securing this position is that, while nobody can claim to have confirmed any such physical lesion or biochemical malfunction as an etiological agent, successes elsewhere with similarly problematic and contested disease hypotheses (e.g., the cases of Alzheimer's discovery of the physical bases of "senile dementia" and of the eventual determination of the neurophysiological anomalies characteristic of "epilepsy") can be invoked to ask for more time before this most recalcitrant of all "psychiatric disorders"--schizophrenia--succumbs (if

---

[3]Miller and Flack (this volume) note that there is empirical evidence to indicate that even between the criteria in the *Diagnostic and Statistical Manual-II* and those in *DSM-III* there have arisen differences significant enough to generate discrepancies in diagnoses such that "research employing the two manuals during the decades when they were used is not comparable. So different is the current version of DSM-III from Bleuler's that Kety (1985) protests, with justification, that the authors should have coined another name in order to avoid confusion with "schizophrenia."

it must) to the verdict of disconfirmation as a genuine disease entity. The problem, then, is familiar one to Popperians: if a scientific theory need only be falsifiable to count as legitimately scientific, how long do critics of any such theory have to wait before its falsification is to be admitted, given the indefinite extendibility of research enterprises predicated upon the *possibility* of its truth?

It seems to me that one solution here is to try to construct an argument designed to show whether or not the continued deployment of a certain way of conceptualizing a problem has become a *barrier* to the effective search for its solution. Can this be done? I believe so, and, a little further on, I will briefly sketch some reasons for this judgment. Before discussing this, however, I would like to interpose some objections to any *generic* skepticism concerning schizophrenia, and to distinguish between two forms of what can be called "social constructionism" in this respect.

Schizophrenia as Social Construction: Two Perspectives

It is notoriously the case that, to many, an argument which asserts that a phenomenon is "socially constructed" is identified as synonymous with an argument which asserts that the phenomenon is an "artifact" of some kind. "Social constructionism" and "realism" in respect of an ontological problem are considered antitheses. Professor Sarbin, for example, tends to assume that a social-constructionist analysis of an object is equivalent to a demonstration of its arbitrariness or non-existence. In elaborating a constructionist thesis, drawing upon the work of Ellard (1987), he points to the nineteenth-century postulate of "masturbatory psychosis" which was eventually abandoned, and implies a similar fate for "schizophrenia."[4] He does not discuss those examples in the history of psychiatry where equally contentious disease assumptions have been sustained, and eventually exonerated, by the discovery of a determinate biological lesion. He also questions the continued use of dopamine blockers following Mesulam's recent skeptical overview of the dopaminergic abnormality hypothesis for schizophrenia (Mesulam, 1990). It seems to me, however, that the evidence in support of the utility of dopamine blockers in transforming or suppressing forms of conduct identified as mentally disordered would have to be assessed *independently* of the

---

[4]One can add the 1975 decision of the U.S. psychiatric profession to delete homosexuality from its catalogue of officially recognized mental disorders.

evidence for and against the dopamine etiological theory for schizophrenia: after all, aspirin reduces fever by inhibiting prostaglandin synthesis, and its utility in doing so is neutral with respect to the issue of whether or not a given fever was caused by the prostaglandins (Creese & Snyder, 1978). Sarbin's position on the social construction of schizophrenia ultimately amounts to a *generalized* form of principled skepticism. "Schizophrenia," he insists, is a myth, an ideology, a metaphorical construction, a "figment of (the psychiatrist's) own disordered consciousness" (quoting Trigant Burrow). So, too, are its putative "symptoms," such as the "hallucinations" variably associated with it: for Sarbin, they are really (socially disvalued) "imaginings."[5]

In assessing objections such as these, it is necessary to recall our initial distinction between assessing the utility of a category like "schizophrenia" for practical, clinical purposes and assessing its utility for theoretical or research purposes. One can distinguish two separable issues here: by treating "schizophrenia" as a *hypothesis* (a concept cannot itself *be* an hypothesis, but it can figure in the construction of an hypothesis, such as: "schizophrenia has a biological/biochemical etiology and may thus be considered a physical disease:" (this need not be its *only* use, however!), and by inferring from failures to confirm a physical basis for the diagnosis to the generic arbitrariness of *any* diagnosis employing the category, Sarbin blurs the fundamental distinction I believe must inform a careful social-constructionist approach to the problem: the differentiation between the clinical and the research domains.[6] We are, if we follow this line of reasoning, left incapable of seeing the concept as it functions within its actual contexts of ascription in the diverse domains where it is used as a basis for various kinds of real-world actions and judgments. Only by resituating the use of the concept within its actual circumstances of consequential usage can we best judge *how* it works—and fails to work—as a device of reasoning and of practical action. Restricting ourselves to reports of reliability studies and of etiological

---

[5]I have questioned this assimilation on conceptual grounds elsewhere (Coulter, 1973; 1975).

[6]It should be remarked here that this distinction is itself a gloss for further possible differentiations that would have to be made by any ethnomethodological inquiry into the social construction of schizophrenia: the clinical domain, for example, easily decomposes into the hospital setting, the incompetency trial setting, the treatment provisions, the case conference setting, record-keeping, and so forth, with their varying personnel. The research domain could encompass circumstances as diverse as the grant application, the theoretical model selection process, the sampling of empirical data, and so forth.

investigations, or to comparisons between generalized descriptions of abstract diagnostic criteria, instructive as these may be for certain purposes, will not bring us any closer to an appreciation of the logic-in-use of the concept of schizophrenia.

A cursory inspection of sociological materials pertaining to the ascription of schizophrenia yields the observation that, contrary to the impression of general arbitrariness, myth-mongering, and purely "ideological" enforcement operations generated by Sarbin's critique, the constitution of a person's status as "schizophrenic" can often be an elaborate social process in which "delusions" are separated from potentially harmless aberrations of belief or subcultural conceptions, "hallucinations" are distinguished from fantasies or misperceptions, and "thought disorder" from confused episodes of conversation or idioms. All of these judgmental operations which inform psychiatric diagnoses are, where they are circumstantially possible at all, predicated upon the exercise of common-sense, situated, logical inquiries into the communicative conduct and contexts of referred persons and locally relevant others. Such judgmental operations require the exercise of a cultural competence which is not the sole prerogative of professional psychiatry, even though it is the clinician who must, in the final analysis, take responsibility for whatever is to be the outcome of the investigative process. Further, while it is true that there are no context-independent, determinate procedures available for ruling *in* a diagnosis of schizophrenia, there are many available procedures for ruling it *out*. If the entire business were quite as arbitrary and power-driven as some critics suggest, why would lay and professional ascribers of schizophrenia tend to take such (routine) trouble to avoid mistakes, conflations with cognate conditions, and unwarranted imputations?

Transformations in the presuppositions informing the use of a category of personal-conduct assessment do not necessarily invalidate every use of such a category. For example, we can still detect melancholia in people despite the fact that we no longer subscribe to the bile theory of the humors (and thus to a *"melange de cholia"*). The absence of algorithmic rules[7] for detecting the presence of a condition or state of affairs does not render us impotent in making

---

[7]Something approximating this ideal was, to my mind, inappropriately demanded by Bleuler (1911/1950) in the articulation of his three criteria for judging whether a proposed syndrome is a discriminable entity as discussed by Miller and Flack (this volume): (1) the category must include symptoms which occur *only and always* in the identified group; (2) no single set of symptoms can be singled out which does not show definite connections or inter-relations with *all* the others, and (3) its criteria can be discovered very easily. (Emphasis mine).

any judgment about its presence or absence; neither does enormous variation in its modes of presentation. For example, being "happy" or being "intelligent" is a state of affairs incapable of being codified into a neat and finite set of behavioral indicators, but we are still fully capable of using those categories in our everyday affairs and dealings with each other. The existence of many borderline cases or of undecidable instances for a given category does not in itself render all of our verdicts useless: some cases may remain quite unambiguous in their contexts of assessment. "Suicide" may be difficult or impossible to distinguish from "accident" on many occasions, but some people can unequivocally be found to have committed it. The fact that the borders of my country may be in dispute does not mean that I can never tell whether I am living there or somewhere else! Absent etiologies do not render all judgments about behavioral or sensory states anomalous or without foundation. The fact that you do not know what is causing the pain in my side does not license you to tell me that I do not have it! The fact that you have no idea what makes me claim (in words and deeds) to be able to see my long-dead brother right now, right in front of me, does not transform my hallucination into a mere exercise of my imagination. If your daughter is genuinely crazy and needs treatment, you are not likely to be assuaged by arguments designed to show that the category of schizophrenia lacks what it lacks: call it "madness," "insanity," "schizophrenia," or whatever you will—she thinks she is Joan of Arc, refuses to go to school and is driving *you* crazy—she needs (medical) *help*, not an epistemological argument. Are we simply settling for inexactness here? As Wittgenstein (1968) observed:

> 'Inexact' is really a reproach, and 'exact' is praise. And that is to say that what is inexact attains its goal less perfectly than what is more exact. Thus the point here is what we call 'the goal.' Am I inexact when I do not give our distance from the sun to the nearest foot, or tell the joiner the width of the table to the nearest thousandth of an inch? No *single* ideal of exactness has been laid down ...

What, then, is the point of adopting a social-constructionist orientation in this field? It is to insist that only by detailing the actual, living interactional processes within which and by which persons come to be categorized as "schizophrenic" can one hope to de-reify our thinking about it as well as exhibit its properties. Such investigations can then furnish genuinely grounded constraints upon theoretical models and philosophical speculations about the phenomena in question. Decontextualizing the "semantics" of the category can only lead to systematic misunderstandings of its functions and the nature of its rules of use.

Bleuler's Concept and Contemporary Etiological Investigations

Nothing in what has been argued so far, however, militates against the adoption of a critical posture toward certain *theoretical* treatments of the phenomena variously grouped under the category of schizophrenia. If I have disagreed with Sarbin in the foregoing, let me hasten to append a fervent agreement with him in his castigation of many current hypotheses and researches based upon stipulative operationalizations of the category and upon inappropriate assumptions about the relationship(s) between biological theorizing and human behavior. Here I shall take up the question of whether or not the continued reliance upon Bleuler's concept of schizophrenia has proven more of a hindrance than a help to etiological investigators.

The first question such an investigator is likely to ask is: how can any etiological inquiry get off the ground if the issue of the very existence of the *explanandum* in question is being rendered problematic? If, as we are told with growing documentation, the category of "schizophrenia" lacks uniform indicators, clear boundaries, common properties, strict recognition rules, or context-independent diagnostic criteria, what is it for which an etiological search is being mounted? Sarbin observes that dependent variables are linked in hypotheses to diagnoses and not to *conduct*. He notes that no causal link is ever postulated in etiological hypotheses between, say, a schizophrenic patient's anomalous brain scan and his specific claims to having daily conversations with the Virgin Mary. We appear stymied even before we enter the research laboratory.

I mentioned earlier some well-intentioned pleas which arose during the conference for the continued deployment of the category of 'schizophrenia' as a heuristic device in psychopathology research projects. I believe that its continuation as a research-guiding construct constitutes a *counter*-heuristic procedure. We do not have to insist that an adequate etiological hypothesis take the form of a postulated link between a genetic, biochemical, or social-psychological dysfunction or anomaly and some very specific belief, perceptual claim, or behavioral orientation on the part of a patient;[8] rather, we should at least insist that the sampling of patients for etiological investigation be governed by an adherence to the rule that they share a range of demonstrably *comparable* properties. That cannot be assured if the sample is generated solely by clinical diagnoses of schizophrenia or of any of its extant sub-types. Premature closure on unreplicated but plausible etiological claims, as well as periodic but unfounded acquiescence in others,[9] is the price that can be, and has been, paid by targeting research upon "schizophrenia."

Conclusion

I have been presenting a case, based upon my assessment of the contributions to this volume, for construing "schizophrenia" not as a simple name for a disease entity with hitherto undiscovered etiology, but as a category which functions in a wider variety of ways: as a device of practical reasoning, as an instrument of professional-clinical adjudication, as a polymorph with ramifying criteria of application, and as a research-guiding construct of dubious utility for generating scientific findings about the bases of problematic forms of human conduct. Since the concept operates differently in diverse language games, attempts to assess its utility must respect such diversity of applications. A failure to appreciate the very different ways in which it enters our lives renders useless attempts to generalize from considerations restricted, e.g., to its purely theoretical utility or lack thereof.

A correct appreciation of the "grammar" of schizophrenia cannot be derived from assessments based upon abstracted renditions housed in DSM-III-R, nor upon depictions insensitive to actual contexts of application. We need better *sociological* elucidations of its grammar of living usage if we are to avoid the twin errors of reification and of conceptual nihilism.

---

[8]For further discussion of some of the problems encountered in specifying the nature of the relationship(s) that obtain between a neural or biochemical phenomenon and a psychological one, see Russell (1984).

[9]For a useful recent discussion of this record, see Lewontin et al. (1984).

References

Angst, J. (1988). European long-term follow up studies of schizophrenia. *Schizophrenia Bulletin, 14*(4), 501-513.

Bentall, R.P. (1986). The scientific status of schizophrenia: A critical evaluation. In N. Eisenberg & G. Glasgow (eds.), *Current issues in clinical psychology*. VT: Croweb.

Bentall, R.P., Jackson, H.F., & Pilgrim, D. (1988). Abandoning the concept of 'schizophrenia': Some implications of validity arguments for psychological research into psychotic phenomena. *British Journal of Clinical Psychology, 27*(4), 303-324.

Bleuler, M. (1911/1950). *Dementia praecox or the group of schizophrenias*. NY: International Universities Press.

Blum, A. (1970). The sociology of mental illness. In Jack D. Douglas (ed.), *Deviance and respectability: The social construction of moral meanings*. N.Y.: Basic Books.

Carpenter, W.T. & Kirkpatrick, B. (1988). The heterogeneity of the long term course of schizophrenia. *Schizophrenia Bulletin*, 14(4), 645-652.

Ciompi, L. (1985). Is there really a schizophrenia? The long-term course of psychotic phenomena. *British Journal of Psychiatry, 146*, 558-559.

Coulter, J. (1975b). Perceptual accounts and interpretive asymmetries. *Sociology, 9*(3), 385-396.

Coulter, J. (1983). *Rethinking cognitive theory*. N.Y.: St. Martin's Press.

Creese, I. & Synder, S.H. (1978). Biochemical investigation: Dopamine. In John C. Shershow (ed.), *Schizophrenia: Science and practice*, p. 148. Cambridge, MA: Harvard University Press.

Cromwell, R.L. (1984). Preemptive thinking and schizophrenia research. In W.D. Spaulding & J.K. Cole (Eds.), *Theories of schizophrenia and psychosis: Nebraska symposium on motivation, 13*. Lincoln, NE: University of Nebraska Press.

Ellard, J. (1987). Did schizophrenia exist before the eighteenth century? *Australian and New Zealand Journal of Psychiatry, 21*(3), 306-314.

Kety, S.S. (1985). The concept of schizophrenia. In M. Alpert (ed.), *Controversies in schizophrenia: Changes and constancies*. N.Y.: Guilford Press.

Lewontin, R.C., Rose, S., & Kamin, L.J. (1984). Schizophrenia: The clash of determinisms. *Not in our genes: Biology, ideology and human nature*. N.Y.: Pantheon Books.

Mesulam, M.M. (1990). Schizophrenia and the brain. *New England Journal of Medicine, 322*(12), 842-845.

Pollner, M. (1974). Sociological and commonsense models of the labeling process. In R. Turner (Ed.), *Ethnomethodology*. Harmondsworth: Penguin.

Pollner, M. (1978). Constitutive and mundane versions of labeling theory. *Human Studies, 1*, 269-288.

Russell, J. (1984). *Explaining mental life*. London: Macmillan.

Scheff, J. (1975). *Labeling madness*. NJ: Prentice-Hall.

Smith, D. (1978). K' is mentally ill. *Sociology, 12*(1), 23-53.

Stephens, J.H. (1982). A comparison of nine systems to diagnose schizophrenia. *Psychiatry Research, 6*(2), 127-143.

Wittgenstein, L. (1968). *Philosophical investigations*. (G.E.M. Anscombe Trans.). Oxford: Basil Blackwell, Oxford).

13

The Social Construction of Schizophrenia[1]

Theodore R. Sarbin

Introduction

In a recent critique of the schizophrenia hypothesis, Bentall, et al. (1988) quote the following paragraph from John Stuart Mill. I borrow the quotation because it aptly conveys the subtext of my analysis:

> The tendency has always been strong to believe that whatever received a name must be an entity or being, having an independent existence of its own. And if no entity answering to the name could be found, men did not for that reason suppose that none existed, but imagined that it was something peculiarly abstruse and mysterious.

Notwithstanding the use of the term "schizophrenia" to denote a firm diagnostic entity by many textbook writers and clinical practitioners, investigators by the hundreds are still trying to establish its empirical validity. The output of published and unpublished research directed toward establishing empirical validity is prodigious, yet schizophrenia remains an unconfirmed hypothesis. The enormous productivity is in the service of breaking out of the pattern of circular reasoning in which "schizophrenia" appears on both sides of a causality equation: absurd behavior betokens the presence of schizophrenia, and schizophrenia is the cause of absurd behavior.

Eugen Bleuler generated the schizophrenia hypothesis to account for certain forms of unwanted conduct. Building on the theories of Emil

[1] I am grateful for helpful suggestions offered by friends and colleagues, among them, Mary Boyle, Ralph M. Carney, William C. Coe, David Cohen, Philip Cowan, Daniel B. Goldstine, Norman S. Greenfield, James C. Mancuso, and Frederick J. Ziegler. An essay based on an earlier version of this paper was published under the title "Toward the obsolescence of the schizophrenia hypothesis" in the *Journal of Mind and Behavior*, 1990.

Kraepelin, he proposed a medical hypothesis—a disease entity—to account for absurd, unwanted conduct. A perusal of standard textbooks in psychiatry and psychology makes clear that the core hypothesis continues to serve as an implicit guide to the construction of current versions of the schizophrenia concept.

In this chapter, I press the claim that I made in other writings (Sarbin, 1969; 1972b; 1990; Sarbin & Mancuso, 1980) that systematic studies have provided no determinate findings to justify continuing the use of schizophrenia-nonschizophrenia as a diagnostic entity. This bold assertion of the failure of the schizophrenia concept should not be interpreted as a challenge to the observation that some people, under some conditions, engage in conduct that others might identify with such terms as crazy, insane, bizarre, mad, irrational, psychotic, deluded, inept, unwanted, or absurd.

"Schizophrenia" is an opaque term. Therefore, scientists and practitioners who employ the term must have some image or accessible prototype when writing their own definitions or formulating a diagnosis. The contemporary construction of schizophrenia was heavily influenced by the prototype advanced by Kraepelin and Bleuler, a prototype exemplified by a person with an infectious brain disease. Because many diagnosed schizophrenics did not fit the specifications of the prototype, some authorities, notably Bleuler, suggested the employment of the plural, "the schizophrenias." This stratagem has not been productive; its main use has been to preserve schizophrenia as a sacred emblem of psychiatry when experiments yielded indeterminate results. A more recent stratagem is the coinage of "schizophrenia spectrum disorders," a category employed to increase the size of an experimental sample in order to achieve statistical significance.

The background for my claim is a personal anthology of the behavior of men and women diagnosed as schizophrenic. Early in my career, I was impressed with the polymorphous nature of the actions of persons who were assigned to the schizophrenia category. In most cases, these actions (I do not prejudge the nature of reported imaginings and expressed beliefs by referring to them as "symptoms") were so specific to the individual's life story that it was difficult for me to accept the lore that some hypothetical brain anomaly could account for the heterogeneity. The notion of a common cause for such an assortment of human actions can be entertained only if, in Procrustean fashion, the interesting array of unwanted actions is reduced to a small number of categories; for example, delusions, flattened affect, and hallucinations; and further, if the categories are redefined as "symptoms" of a still-to-be-discovered disease entity. Such a redefinition turns attention away from the problem-solving features of each person's conduct. Most important, the redefinition renders irrelevant the search for intentions and meanings behind perplexing interpersonal acts.

The Scientific Search for Diacritica

It was in the early 1960s that I undertook seriously to question the lore that had grown up around the schizophrenia concept. I followed two strategies: the first was to determine the epistemic and social pathways leading from particular actions of putative patients to diagnostic judgments by mental health professionals; the second was to determine from a search of the published experimental literature whether a stable set of referents had been discovered that would validate the schizophrenia hypothesis.

I chose to study hallucinations (reported imaginings) and delusions (atypical beliefs) and how diagnosticians employed these categories in constructing a diagnosis of schizophrenia. After working several years in the clinic and in the laboratory to understand hallucination and delusion, I concluded that the epistemic process of constructing imaginings and beliefs was the same for so-called schizophrenics and so-called normals (Sarbin, 1967; 1972a; Juhasz & Sarbin, 1966; Sarbin & Juhasz, 1982; 1978; 1975; 1970; 1967). The technical and pejorative terms "hallucination" and "delusion" were selectively assigned by clinicians to devalued or degraded persons as symptoms of disease. In most instances, those who employed these terms were not concerned with fathoming the meanings of such behaviors or the part these behaviors played in the patient's life story. Among the exceptions to this generalization is a study reported by Benjamin (1989). In a carefully crafted investigation she demonstrated that the auditory hallucinations of psychiatric patients were meaningful and reflected widely observed interpersonal themes. Further, the "voices" appeared to have an important adaptive function for the patients.

The second strategy in my search was to determine to what extent, if any, the published research could be used to support the schizophrenia hypothesis. It was not unreasonable to suppose that the schizophrenia hypothesis must have some validity because so much journal space was devoted to experimental studies. In the early 1970s, I made some casual forays into the experimental literature, looking for support for then-popular theories of schizophrenia. My preliminary analysis made clear that most of the theories of schizophrenia had been initially supported on the basis of one or two experiments. When replicated by other investigators, the results of these experiments proved to be artifacts. Each theory had a short period of enthusiastic support and then a marked decline.

In addition to theories proposing psychological variables, a large number of theories called for the assessment of biochemical substances, on the assumption that the perplexing actions of schizophrenics were caused by irregularities in brain chemistry. The strategy was to look for markers in blood or urine samples. A series of observations (Hoffer & Mahon, 1961; Hoffer & Osmond, 1963) led to the identification of the "mauve spot" in the chromatographs of the urine of hospitalized patients. Other investigators subsequently noted that the mauve spot disappeared when neuroleptic medication was withdrawn. This biochemical theory of schizophrenia lost its credibility when the marker, the mauve spot, was found to be a metabolite of the medication designed to control patient behavior.

The rise and fall of these and other theories led me to conclude that both somatic and psychological theories of schizophrenia have a half-life of about five years.

In a more systematic analysis of the published literature, Professor James Mancuso and I reviewed every research article on schizophrenia published in the *Journal of Abnormal Psychology*[2] for the 20-year period beginning in 1959 (Sarbin & Mancuso, 1980). We selected this journal because of its high standards, the average manuscript rejection rate being about 80 percent. (To fend off any criticism that we had introduced a bias in selecting a psychological journal, we appended to our analysis a review of selected articles from psychiatric journals.) We found 374 reports of experiments in the *Journal*. By any standard, the published psychological research on schizophrenia during the 20-year period represented a prodigious effort. It is abundantly clear that in the period under review, students of deviant conduct focused on the central problem: identifying a reliable diagnostic marker, psychological or somatic, that would replace subjective (and fallible) diagnosis. The discovery of such a marker would establish the long sought-for validity for the postulated entity, schizophrenia (and, co-incidentally, would make the investigator a prime candidate for a Nobel Prize).

In nearly all the studies, schizophrenia/nonschizophrenia was the independent variable. To accomplish their mission, investigators compared the mean responses of "schizophrenics" on experimental tasks with the mean responses of persons who were not so diagnosed. It is no exaggeration to say that the experimental tasks devised by creative investigators numbered in the hundreds. All were constructed

---

[2]Until 1964, *Journal of Abnormal and Social Psychology*.

for the purpose of rigorously testing miniature hypotheses linked to the postulate that schizophrenia was an identifiable mental disease or disorder. The experimental hypotheses were formulated with the expectation that whatever the task, schizophrenics would, on the average, perform poorly when compared with the average performance of a control group. When we look at the range and variety of the experimental tasks, it becomes apparent at once that the formulators of these experimental hypotheses shared the conviction that "schizophrenics" were persons who were basically flawed; they believed that the putative disease affected all somatic and psychological systems. It was as if all the experimenters had absorbed Kraepelin's dictum:

> We designate as dementia praecox the development of a simple, more or less pervasive, state of mental weakness, which manifests itself as an acute or subacute mental disorder. The course of this disease process can exhibit very different patterns ... [I]n all likelihood we are dealing with an organic change in the brain (1908, p. 125).

Mancuso and I analyzed the 374 studies on several dimensions. Among the conclusions we drew was that the criteria for selecting subjects were less than satisfactory. The typical study gave short shrift to the manners in which the subjects, mental hospital patients, were selected. The unreliability of psychiatric diagnosis notwithstanding, the experimenters were satisfied to accept diagnoses made by "two staff psychiatrists," "by a psychiatrist and a psychologist," "by consensus in diagnostic staff conference," etc. It is unknown to what extent the diagnosticians employed the second edition of the *Diagnostic and Statistical Manual*, although it is likely that the lore contained in the *Manual* provided the diagnostic criteria.[3] The dependent variables were assessed with great precision, sometimes to two decimal places. In contrast, the independent variable, schizophrenia/nonschizophrenia, was assessed either by the subjective and fallible judgments of clinicians, or by a vote taken in a diagnostic staff conference.

To bring our analysis up to date, we performed the same analysis on the reports published in the *Journal of Abnormal Psychology* for the ten year period, 1979-1988. It was in this period that DSM-III and

---

[3] The constantly changing criteria for schizophrenia in the various editions of the *Diagnostic and Statistical Manual* render it well-nigh impossible to aggregate the results of research studies. Blum (1978) compared diagnostic practices in 1954, 1964, and 1974 in the same hospital. About one-third of persons diagnosed as schizophrenic in 1954 would acquire a different diagnosis 20 years later.

DSM-III-R came into use. During this period structured interviews were developed to increase the reliability of diagnosis. Scientists expected that these systematic aids to diagnosis would facilitate the discovery of valid markers for schizophrenia. Our examination of the research reports shows that the experiments reported during the period 1979-1988 followed the same pattern that we had discerned in the earlier analysis. The Kraepelinian premise that schizophrenics are basically flawed organisms continues to guide the formulation of research hypotheses (Sarbin, Mancuso, & Podczerwinski, in preparation).

About 80% of the studies reported that schizophrenics performed poorly when compared to control subjects. Variability in performance was the rule. Although the published studies reported that mean differences between groups were statistically significant, the differences were very small. In those studies where it was possible to reconstruct distributions, it was immediately clear that the performances of the schizophrenic samples and the normal samples overlapped considerably. An examination of a number of such distributions points to an unmistakable conclusion: most schizophrenics cannot be differentiated from most normals on a wide variety of experimental tasks. If one were to employ the dependent variable as a marker for schizophrenia in a new sample, the increase in diagnostic accuracy would be infinitesimal.

In two of the studies, the mean scores of the schizophrenic sample —contrary to expectations—were superior to the mean scores of the control sample. Such results violate the generally accepted notion that schizophrenics are basically flawed. In these experiments, the schizophrenic subjects followed the task instructions better than the controls. The investigators resolved the resulting dissonance by the post hoc explanation that the schizophrenics interpreted the task instructions too literally (Broen & Nakamura, 1972; Thornton & Gottheil, 1971). The explanation served to save the schizophrenia hypothesis—after all, is not literalness a sign of thought disorder?

That so many studies showed small mean differences has been taken to mean that the schizophrenia hypothesis has earned a modicum of credibility. This credibility dissolves when we consider a number of hidden variables that could account for the observed differences. A large number of reports noted that the schizophrenic subjects were on neuroleptic medication. It is appropriate to ask whether the small mean differences could be accounted for by the drugged status of the experimental subjects and the non-drugged status of the controls. Other hidden variables are socioeconomic status and education. Since at least 1855, it has been noted that the diagnosis of insanity (later dementia praecox and schizophrenia) has been employed primarily as a diagnosis for poor people (Dohrenwend, 1990). Many of the experimental tasks called for cognitive skills. The mean difference in performance on such tasks could well be related to cognitive skills, a correlate of education and socioeconomic status. Some experimenters noted the difficulty in recruiting control subjects whose educational level matched the low levels of schizophrenics who in many instances had more than a tenth-grade education.

Not assessed in these studies were the effects of patienthood. At the time the hospitalized patients were recruited to be subjects, they had been the objects of legal, medical, nursing, and, in some cases, police procedures, not to mention mental hospital routines and their effects on personal identity. As mentioned before, only cooperative, i.e., docile, patients are recruited. It would be instructive to investigate to what degree docility influences the subjects' approach to the experimental tasks.

Any of the hidden variables could account for the small mean differences observed in experimental studies. One conclusion is paramount: the 30 years of psychological research covered in our analyses yielded no marker that would establish the validity of the schizophrenia construct.

The argument could be made that psychological variables are too crude to identify the disease process. Some would argue (e.g., Meehl, 1989), that biochemical, neurological, and anatomical studies are more likely to reveal the ultimate marker for schizophrenia. Other contributors to this book, e.g., Zubin, McHugh, and Kendell, argue that the extensive research on eye-movements, brain morphology, and electrophysiology have firmly established the ontological basis for schizophrenia.

The research and theoretical contributions of proponents of the biological etiology of schizophrenia may be viewed as instances of scientific claims-making. The claim is that schizophrenia is a biomedical disease. Proponents support their beliefs by pointing to extensive research (aided by high technology) on brain morphology, electrophysiology, and brain chemistry. In the typical study, diagnosed schizophrenics are compared with medical patients or normal controls. In recent years, size of the cerebral ventricles has been studied extensively. The typical study concludes that the size of the ventricles of schizophrenic patients is larger than that of the ventricles of control subjects. The phenomenon of oversized ventricles has been given a proper name: ventriculomegaly. The conclusions are drawn from comparisons of *mean* differences. To calculate a mean requires that assessments of the ventricle size be homogenized, along with the assessments of the contrast groups. Because most of the studies were performed to find a valid marker for schizophrenia, it would be appropriate to report the proportions of schizophrenics whose ventricles were within the "normal" range and also the proportion of the control subjects with enlarged ventricles. If size of cerebral ventricles were to be employed as a replacement for clinical diagnosis, an unacceptable number of normals would be diagnosed as schizophrenic and an unacceptable number of schizophrenics would be diagnosed as normal. In a meta-analysis of almost 100 published studies on brain abnormalities in which high technology imaging techniques were employed, Raz and Raz (1990) concluded that ventriculomegaly in schizophrenia is a reliable phenomenon. They added the qualification: "Although the enlargement of the ventricles observed in schizophrenia may be viewed by the radiologist as only mild compared with pathological conditions involving obstruction of CSF flow, it nonetheless corresponds to 37-43% nonoverlap between the distributions of schizophrenic and control subjects" (p. 102).

This careful meta-analysis reveals the epistemological assumptions underlying biomedical and psychological research. The use of significance tests to establish confidence in group differences can indicate only that the null hypothesis is unsupported. The degree of non-overlap is taken as support for the theoretical hypothesis. That more than half (57-63%) of the subjects cannot be differentiated into schizophrenia/nonschizophrenia ought to direct investigators to explore the sources of variation, one of which could be the heterogeneity of the schizophrenic samples. One failing of this genre of research is the emphasis on seeking connections between *diagnoses* and brain pathology rather than *behavior* and brain pathology. The closest approximation to employing a behavior index is examining the length of "cumulative hospitalization."[4] The correlation between effect size and cumulative hospitalization (controlled for age and "length of illness") accounted for no more than 21% of the variance.

In reviewing biomedical studies, I was impressed with the similarity of the epistemological assumptions made by researchers looking for psychological markers and by researchers seeking biological markers. Both employ significance tests to determine whether the observed differences could be attributed to chance. The epistemological assumption is that a significance test (e.g., $p < .01$) is a warrant for truth when in fact it is only a probability estimate for rejecting the null hypothesis.

In reviewing the morphological and electrophysiological studies, nearly all of which report differences that they claim are associated

---

[4]We can put aside the fact that such an index might tell us more about the behavior of spouses, parents, and doctors than about the patient.

with schizophrenia, I found no instance in which confidence in the claim resulted in the investigators' recommendation that the biological marker be substituted for clinical diagnosis.

I do not discount the importance of biomedical findings and their contribution to understanding brain functioning. It is a long leap of faith, however, to hold that eye-movement distortions, brain wave anomalies, or degree of ventriculomegaly is related to the presence or absence of absurd conduct. What has not been demonstrated is a relationship between say, ventriculomegaly, and the presence or absence of a belief in leprechauns, ineptness in social relations, or a claim to hear non-existent voices. Hardly considered by biomedical investigators is the relationship between a putative marker and changing behavior patterns over time. The heterogeneity of the course and outcome of "schizophrenia" is well established (Carpenter & Kirkpatrick, 1988). If the patient improves, does the size of the cerebral ventricles change?[5] It is important to note the high degree of variability in biomedical and psychological measurements. To isolate the elusive marker, investigators must discover indicators that cluster near the mean for the experimental sample and at the same time do not overlap with the control sample or with other presumed diagnostic entities. None of the published psychological or biomedical studies meet this requirement.

Constructing Schizophrenia

Although the prevailing mechanistic framework directs practitioners to perceive crazy behavior as ultimately caused by anatomical or biochemical anomalies, I suggest a different perspective. I begin from the observation that the candidates for the diagnosis of schizophrenia are not people who seek out doctors for the relief of pain or discomfort. Rather, they are persons who undergo a pre-diagnostic phase in which moral judgments are made on their nonconforming or perplexing actions by family members, employers, police officers, or neighbors. In the absence of reliable tests to demonstrate that the unwanted conduct was caused by anatomical or biochemical

---

[5]My critique of the studies purporting to show that cerebral pathology bears a causal relation to schizophrenia could be applied *in toto* to studies of eye-movement dysfunction. Although proponents of the disease construction cite low level correlations, the relationship between conduct that leads to a diagnosis of schizophrenia and eye movement dysfunctions is not settled. In an in-depth methodological review, Clementz and Sweeney (1990) concluded that the reported findings are "promising," but "their significance for elucidating the diagnostic bandwidth, pathophysiology, and genetics ... remains to be determined" (p. 77).

distortions, diagnosticians unwittingly join in the moral enterprise. They confirm the initial pre-diagnostic judgment that the deviant behavior belongs to a class of unwanted behaviors. After appropriate rituals they confirm the moral verdict and encode it with a proper medical term—schizophrenia.

The foregoing remarks are preliminary to my argument that schizophrenia is a social construction initially put forth as a hypothesis by medical scientists and practitioners. A social construction is an organized set of beliefs that has the potential to guide action. The construction is communicated, elaborated and negotiated by means of linguistic and rhetorical symbols and organizational acts. Like any construction, the schizophrenia hypothesis serves certain purposes and not others.

To find the origin of the schizophrenia construction, one must refer to historical sources. Because of space limitations, I must forgo a full historical account and instead point to some pertinent observations.

Ellard (1987), an Australian psychiatrist, has contributed a provocative argument under the title "Did schizophrenia exist before the eighteenth century?" His historical analysis begins from a skeptical posture, namely, to "reflect on the question whether or not there has ever been an entity of any kind at all that stands behind the word, 'schizophrenia,' and if so, what its true nature might be." Citing well-known authorities, Ellard points to significant changes in the description of schizophrenia over the past 50 or 60 years. He cites the common observation that contemporary clinicians seldom encounter patients who fit the prototypes advanced by Kraepelin and Bleuler. If the nosological criteria for schizophrenia has changed so radically in a half-century, is it not conceivable that the criteria changed significantly in the half-century before Kraepelin and Bleuler? and in the half-century before that?[6]

---

[6]It appears that the rate of change in the criteria for schizophrenia is accelerating. In less than a decade, two revisions of the *Diagnostic and Statistical Manual* appeared. DSM-III was published in 1980 and DSM-III-R in 1987. A new revision, DSM-IV, is in the offing. These *Manuals* are products of consensual judgments by psychiatric experts nominated by task forces of the American Psychiatric Association. In the 1970s, the Present State Examination (PSE) was developed in England for making diagnoses and implemented by a computer system (Wing et al., 1974). The criteria in the PSE were taken from Schneider (1959) who, for example, regarded certain "hallucinations" as "first-rank" symptoms. The earlier editions of the American Manual had adapted Bleuler's four "A's" as criteria (anhedonia, associations, ambivalence, and autism) and looked upon "hallucinations" as accessory, not central, phenomena. More recent editions are neo-Kraepelinian—hallucinations and delusions are categorized as psychotic phenomena. The overlap between the two systems is far from perfect; each selects different candidates for what appear to be the same diagnostic categories. van den Brink et al. (1989) compared the two systems on an outpatient psychiatric population. The two systems converged on 115 of 175 patients, yielding a kappa coefficient of .32.

As a point of departure, Ellard takes the construction and eventual abandonment of the nineteenth-century diagnosis, masturbatory psychosis. Medical orthodoxy posited a psychosis characterized by restlessness, silliness, intellectual deterioration, and inappropriate affect. The entrenched belief in the association between biological activities and crazy behavior nurtured the idea of masturbatory insanity well into the twentieth century. Although at one time professionally acceptable, it was ultimately abandoned as an empty, if not counterproductive, diagnosis.

Employing the vaguely defined "thought disorder" as the criterion for schizophrenia, Ellard searched the literature for evidence of cases noted by physicians and historians. His reading of case histories and medical records led to the conclusion that insanities involving "thought disorders" were identified in the eighteenth and nineteenth centuries, but such cases were exceedingly rare in the seventeenth century. It remains for future historians to identify the social, political, and professional conditions that brought about the creation of a diagnosis centered on ambiguously defined "thought disorder."[7]

Ellard's observation about the changing criteria for schizophrenia receives strong support from a historical analysis prepared by Boyle (1990), in which she advances a convincing explanation for the changing symptoms. Like Ellard, Boyle cites the well-documented observation that the kind of deteriorated cases described by Kraepelin and Bleuler are rarely, if ever, seen in modern times. Kraepelin recorded somatic signs and symptoms of some of his dementia praecox patients that were consistent with his gloomy prognosis of outcome: "marked peculiarities of gait..., excess production of saliva, and urine; dramatic weight fluctuations; tremor; cyanosis of the hands and feet; constraint of movement and the inability, in spite of effort, to complete 'willed' acts." Kraepelin also reported brain damage as revealed microscopically at post-mortem. Bleuler noted similar phenomena; for example, he claimed to be able to diagnose a schizophrenic by his gait.

When Kraepelin and Bleuler were establishing the diagnoses of dementia praecox and schizophrenia, they had no way of knowing that their patient populations might have included a sizable number of persons suffering from post-encephalitic parkinsonism or other organic

---

[7]The origins of the antecedents to the schizophrenia diagnosis occurred about the same time as the construction of the notion of the modern nuclear family (Gubrium & Holstein, 1990). The most frequent path to the mental hospital are the complaints of family members. These observations might lead a historical researcher to take a fresh look at family communications hypotheses such as those advanced by Bateson et al. (1956), Singer and Wynne (1963), and others.

anomalies. It was not until 1917 that the Austrian neurologist, Von Economo, identified encephalitis lethargica, popularly known as sleeping sickness. The sequelae to the infection include post-encephalitic parkinsonism, signs and symptoms very much like the signs and symptoms that Kraepelin had noted for dementia praecox. A number of encephalitis epidemics had swept through Europe, culminating in the epidemic of 1916-1927. Before von Economo's identification of encephalitis lethargica, persons presenting themselves to clinics and hospitals with the symptoms of post-encephalitic parkinsonism could be tagged with any number of diagnoses, including dementia praecox.

Modern-day psychiatrists and psychologists do not encounter crazy patients who fit Kraepelin's and Bleuler's descriptions; that is, patients who display the features of post-encephalitic parkinsonism or other organic conditions. The change in symptoms over the past 50 or 75 years, then, is the result of not including encephalitic patients in the pool of patients who come to the attention of mental health professionals.

Boyle's historical account lends credibility to the thesis that post-encephalitic parkinsonism was unwittingly employed as the model for dementia praecox and schizophrenia. Thus the social construction of schizophrenia as a form of mental disease was facilitated by erroneously sorting two types of persons into a single class: undiagnosed post-encephalitic (or other organic) patients, and persons who had engaged in various kinds of unwanted conduct. The latter, who presented conduct only superficially similar to brain-damaged individuals, were assimilated to the former.

The Medicalization of Madness

Two features sustain the vitality of any social construction: the utility of the construction in solving certain societal problems; and the support it receives from authoritative sources and from the force of concurrent ideological commitments.

1. Social Utility of the Schizophrenia Construction

The social construction of schizophrenia was elaborated in the context of the asylum movement. The history of the nineteenth-century asylum movement makes clear how madness was medicalized. In the ferment produced by rapid progress in all branches of science and technology, madness became a fit subject for scientific work. It was in the nineteenth century that medical practitioners introduced a host of new diagnoses (Rosenberg, 1989). When called upon to deal with crazy people, in the spirit of the rapidly advancing medical sciences, they formulated new diagnoses, among them, dementia praecox.

Asylums became mental hospitals, institutions that filled a number of societal needs, the most salient of which was social control—the maintenance of order. A cursory glance at the treatments introduced over the past 150 years demonstrates clearly the operation of a mechanistic (read medical) ideology to solve the problem of control. Locked wards and physical restraints were supplemented with treatments that were manifestly medical. Bloodletting and emetics, relics of Galenic theory, were widely practiced and ultimately abandoned. Treatments that were consistent with developing medical theories were invented; among them, unlimited surgery to rid the patient's body of focal infections. Scull (1987) has written a Gothic horror tale of the focal infection theory and the unwarranted surgery practiced by dentists and surgeons in their efforts to control unwanted conduct. Enthusiasm for such treatments went unchecked until it became public knowledge that the high mortality rates could not justify the small number of patients whose behavior was brought under control. The more recent history of insulin, metrazol, and electroshock therapies provide additional support for the claim that social control was the object of the therapies. Frontal lobotomy as a means of behavior control was another surgical treatment based on the entrenched belief that unwanted conduct was somehow caused by malfunctioning frontal lobes (Valenstein, 1986). Just a short time ago, biologically-oriented psychiatrists, influenced by the same ideology, employed hemodialysis in an effort to rid patients of the presumed schizotoxin.

The most recent application of this ideology is the attempt to control behavior through the use of neuroleptic medications.   The justification for the prescription of such medications is the dopamine hypothesis, that schizophrenic behavior is the result of an excess of dopaminergic activity. Phenothiazine medications block such activity and, in some patients, there is a diminution of unacceptable activity. However, it has been observed that there is not only a reduction of unacceptable behavior, but also of other activities. The behavior control brought about by the medications has its price, however. Structural and histological damage to the brain is known to follow the prolonged use of phenothiazines. Tardive dyskinesia has been observed in a substantial proportion of patients (Breggin, 1983; Cohen, 1989; Cohen & Cohen, 1986). Contemporary clinical practice, however, accepts the notion that dopamine blockers are the medications of choice. The rationale for prescribing dopamine blockers is questioned in a recent editorial in the prestigious *New England Journal of Medicine:* "Despite a number of suggestive findings,...there is currently no proof that either a neurotoxin or an abnormality of transmission (including a dopaminergic abnormality) is a primary feature of schizophrenia" (Mesulam, 1990).

Clearly, the schizophrenia construction has been useful to mental health practitioners; it has provided a justification for diagnosis. The availability of the diagnostic term, schizophrenia, like the availability of its superordinate, mental illness, is useful as a step in the societal process of controlling persons whose conduct is unacceptable to others. Since the development of the profession of medicine and especially the discipline of psychiatry, the control of patient conduct has for the most part been accomplished by means of traditional medical procedures: surgery and medication. I have identified a few of these procedures. All had their moment in the sun and were later discarded when proven to be ineffective or harmful. During the period that each of the procedures was considered professionally ethical and potentially effective, however, the time-honored sequence "first diagnosis, then treatment" gave illusory support to the construal of unwanted conduct as a disease process.

In many cases, the act of diagnosing was no more than a ritual exercise because of the ignorance of the effects of available treatments and the remote outcomes of these treatments. Psychiatric diagnosing has become increasingly dependent on published manuals. The importance given to the development of diagnostic manuals appears to be out of proportion to their utility. The obsessive preoccupation with diagnosis is illustrated in the history of the *Diagnostic and Statistical Manual.* Blashfield et al. (1990) have noted that the first *Diagnostic and Statistical Manual,* published in 1952, contained 106 categories, the second, published in 1968, contained 182, the third, published in 1980, contained 265, and the fourth, published in 1987 (DSM-III-R), contained 292. "By linear extrapolation, the DSM-IV should be expected to contain about 350 categories ..." This progression points to the arbitrary nature of the process of including or excluding diagnostic categories.

In his study of almost 11,000 patients in a university teaching hospital, Loranger (1990) noted the marked reduction in the use of "schizophrenia" when DSM-III criteria displaced DSM-II criteria. Twice as many patients had been tagged with the schizophrenia label in the DSM-II period (1975-1980) when compared with diagnoses assigned during the DSM-III period (1980-1985).

2. Legitimization of the Construal of Schizophrenia

Despite its failure when examined by empirical methods, the social construction of schizophrenia has persisted because it has been supported in various ways. Two classes of support can be identified: support intrinsic to the biomedical model; and support extrinsic to the model in the form of social practices and unarticulated beliefs.

Biological research has served as a means of intrinsic support for the schizophrenia construction. I need only mention the names of some of the hypotheses that have been subjected to laboratory and clinical testing; taraxein, CPK (creatine phosphokinase), serotonin, dopamine, ventriculomegaly. The composite effect of all this research activity has been to create the belief that an entity exists, waiting for refined methods and high technology to identify the causal morphological, neuro-transmission, or biochemical factor. As I indicated before, countless studies have not identified the disease entity in any determinate way. Rhapsodic response greeted each report of a brain anomaly, toxin, or biochemical abnormality, although the more cautious reviewers would assert only that the variables "had promise." Nevertheless, the profession and the public have interpreted the sustained research activity by responsible scientists as evidence that the schizophrenia construction is a tenable one.

In addition to direct biological research, the genetic transmission hypothesis has been advanced to support the construction of schizophrenia. Highly visible scientists have reported a heritability factor for schizophrenia. Wide publicity, both within the profession and outside, has been given to studies of twins and to studies of children of schizophrenics who were reared by adoptive parents (See, for example, Gottesman & Shields, 1972; Kety, Rosenthal, Wender, & Shulsinger, 1968; Kety, Rosenthal, Wender, Shulsinger, & Jacobsen, 1975). Current textbooks cite these investigations as revealed truth, but the extensive critiques of the studies are seldom noted. That the reported studies are riddled with methodological, statistical and interpretational errors has been repeatedly demonstrated (See especially, Abrams & Taylor, 1983; Benjamin, 1976; Kringlen & Cramer, 1989; Lewontin, Kamin, & Rose, 1984; Lidz, 1990; Lidz & Blatt, 1983; Lidz, Blatt, & Cook, 1981; Marshall, 1986; Sarbin & Mancuso, 1980). The extent of these criticisms suggests that establishing the validity of "schizophrenia" should have had logical priority over the identification of its genetic features.

My thesis holds for genetic research as it does for psychological and biological research: no firm ontological basis has been established for schizophrenia. In the absence of determinate criteria, investigators direct their efforts toward discovering intergenerational similarities

—not of identifiable behavior—but of *diagnoses*, a far cry from behavioral genetics, in which intergenerational similarities of *behavior* are studied.[8]

In addition to intrinsic supports, it is possible to identify a number of extrinsic supports that help explain the tenacity of the schizophrenia construction. Although constructions that are congruent with the concurrent scientific paradigm may appear to be self-supporting, they are sustained in great measure by forces external to the scientific enterprise.

A vast network of government bureaucracies legitimize biomedical conceptions of deviant conduct, including schizophrenia. Federal agencies that control research grants advocate studies that aim to understand and ultimately control "the dread disease." The National Institutes of Health has promoted the schizophrenia construction in many ways, including the sponsorship of the *Schizophrenia Bulletin*.

The power of bureaucracy would be minimal if its implicit messages about schizophrenia fell on deaf ears. A readiness to believe the schizophrenia story follows from the unwitting acceptance of an ideology—a network of historically conditioned premises.

Ideology carries the meaning that knowledge is situationally determined—the worldview and the social status of the scientist influence the content of knowledge. An examination of ideological premises illuminates how an entrenched professional organization can become so bound to a situation that its members cannot recognize facts that would dissolve the power of the organization. An ideology has a sacred quality. A challenge to a claim based on ideological premises usually invokes passionate, rather than reasoned, responses. Note the heated responses to the writings of Szasz, Laing, Rosenhan, and other critics of the official schizophrenia doctrine.

Hays (1984), commenting on the inclusion of a polymorphous set of behaviors in one nosological class, succinctly addressed the role of ideology.

> Medicine is a conservative profession. What doctors know is passed on to students. In this way they honestly associate themselves with their own body of knowledge and as responsible guarantors of its truth. It is natural for such men and women to shy away from radical formulations which threaten their hard-won data-base, introduce uncertainty, and

---

[8]Kety, one of the leading advocates of the genetic transmission hypothesis, wrote a critique of Rosenhan's famous study (1973) "Being Sane in Insane Places." In the critique, he composed a rhetorical sentence that lends itself to a literal interpretation: "If schizophrenia is a myth, it is a myth with a very strong genetic component" (1974).

reduce the worth of what they have learned and what they have to offer. The presentation of a conceptualization which is at variance with extant schemata may be received as an affront ... It is hard, therefore, to envisage how even the most tactful and elaborate preamble can render palatable the proposition that ... schizophrenia does not exist. (p. 5)

One strand in the texture of the ideology of schizophrenia is the institution of the mental hospital. The transformation of the asylum into a mental hospital, in the context of preserving order, paved the way for regarding inmates as objects. Because of the culturally enscripted roles for physicians and patients, once the physician made the diagnosis, the patient became a figure in an altered social narrative. The power of physicians over patients created a condition in which physicians could distance themselves from patients—a necessary precondition for the draconian surgical and medical treatments mentioned previously.[9]

The legitimate power of the physician remains an unquestioned premise in the social construction of schizophrenia as a disease entity. But legitimate power is only one of the characteristics silently assumed in the course of physicians enacting their roles. Physicians carry Aesculapian authority, an authority that supplements legitimate power with moral and charismatic authority (Siegler & Osmund, 1973). They are assumed to have moral power because of their dedication to relieving pain and curing illness. Since religious figures once participated in healing activities, physicians are also assumed to have the charisma that goes with the priestly role. Aesculapian authority continues to operate as a silent premise for government bodies that allocate funds in support of research the aim of which is the control of crazy people.[10]

---

[9]It is instructive to trace the emphasis on diagnosis to its historical roots. Craik (1959) revived the historical notion that the early Greeks recognized that different outcomes were entailed if the doctor emphasized the *disease* or the *person*. The focus on diagnosing and treating the disease is associated with a school of medical practice on the island of Cnidus. A contrary view is associated with Hippocrates of Cos. The Cosan view recognized the necessity of dealing with the whole patient—his illness in relation to biography. The doctor-patient script was a collaborative one. The prevailing ideology in medicine, including psychiatry, is Cnidian. The doctor-patient script diminished the role of biography in therapy. In their research, psychologists have borrowed the Cnidian point of view. They begin the research enterprise with subjects who have been "diagnosed" as schizophrenic, thus embracing—sometimes unwittingly—the disease construction. Once the diagnosis is made, the life-narrative of the patient is irrelevant.

[10]In the interest of brevity, I have omitted a discussion of several other premises that undergird the social construction of schizophrenia. These are described in Sarbin and Mancuso (1980).

A parallel premise is that "certain types of people are more dangerous than other types of people" (Sarbin and Mancuso, 1980). The origin of the connection between being schizophrenic and being dangerous is obscure. Several strands in the fabric of this premise can be identified, among them, the Calvinistic equation of being poor with being damned, and the attribution of "dangerous classes" to the powerless poor.

The overrepresentation of poor people in the class "schizophrenics" has been repeatedly documented. In addition, Pavkov, Lewis, and Lyons (1989) have shown that both being black and coming to the attention of mental health professionals is predictive of a diagnosis of schizophrenia. Recently, Landrine (1989) has concluded on the basis of research evidence that the social role of poor people is a stereotype in the epistemic structure of middle-class diagnosticians. The linguistic performances and social interactions of poor people have the same quality as the performances of men and women diagnosed as schizophrenics, particularly those schizophrenics of the "negative type" (Andreasen, 1982), social failures who have adopted a strategy of minimal action.[11]

The translation from the expression of atypical, unassimilable conduct (craziness) to being dangerous is facilitated by the myth of the "wild man within." The distinguished historian, Hayden White (1972), has described how the myth grew out of beliefs held by Europeans during times when unknown lands were being discovered. Because the inhabitants of exotic places engaged in conduct that differed so markedly from Western norms, Europeans looked upon such people as being unsocialized, untamed, wild savages. The world (which seems to be continually shrinking) has unearthed no wild man of Borneo or of any other place, but the myth of the "wild man within" lingers as an unspoken basis for attributing dangerousness to crazy people. The myth found expression and, *a fortiori*, support in

---

[11]It is interesting to note that with the revived emphasis on the Kraepelinian construction, interest in studying the relations between socio-economic status (SES) and psychiatric diagnoses has declined. This decline in interest is not due to any change in the facts. Schizophrenia is primarily a diagnosis for poor people. The advent of neo-Kraepelinian models, especially the diathesis-stress construction, turned attention to genetics and to the study of stress. But SES has not figured prominently in stress research. Dohrenwend (1989), a leading epidemiologist, has noted that "...relations between SES or social class and psychiatric disorders have provided the most challenging cues to the role of adversity in the development of psychiatric disorders. The problem remains what it has always been: how to unlock the riddle that low SES can be either a cause or a consequence of psychopathology." The adversity thesis might be illuminated through an examination of the observation that the outcome of "schizophrenia" varies with economic and social conditions (Warner, 1985).

Landrine's research, cited above, adds to the puzzle another dimension: lower-class stereotypes held by middle-class diagnosticians.

Lombroso's notion of "atavism" and Freud's concept of the impulse-ridden Id.[12]

The Futility of the Mechanistic Paradigm in Human Affairs

The concept of schizophrenia originated out of the need to deal with people whose conduct was not acceptable to others who were more powerful. During the hey-day of nineteenth-century science, the construction was guided by metaphors drawn from mechanistic biology. Physicians formulated their theories and practices from constructions that grew out of developing knowledge in anatomy, chemistry, and physiology. The construction had an ideological cast—its proponents were blind to the possibilities that the absurdities[13] exhibited by mental hospital patients were efforts at sense-making. Instead, they followed the tenets of mechanistic science: that social misconduct, like rashes, fevers, aches, pains, and other somatic conditions, is caused by disease processes.

Reliable and sustained empirical evidence—a cardinal requirement of mechanistic science—has not been put forth to validate the schizophrenia hypothesis. Despite the absence of empirical support, the schizophrenia construction continues its tenacious hold on theory and practice.

My recommendation is that we banish schizophrenia to the dustbin of history along with other previously valued scientific constructions; among them, phlogiston, the luminiferous ether, the geocentric view of the universe; and closer to home, monomania, neurasthenia, masturbatory insanity, lycanthropy, demon possession, and mopishness.

I emphasize that I am not recommending formulating a new descriptive term to replace schizophrenia. The referents for schizophrenia are too diverse, confounded, changing, and ambiguous (Carpenter & Kirkpatrick, 1988). The fact that two (or 200) persons who exhibit no absurdities in common may be tagged with the same label demonstrates the vacuity of the concept.

In the body of my text, I asserted that the harvest from the traditional approach—derived from the mechanistic metaphysic—has

---

[12]An advertisement in one of the psychiatric journals continues the rhetorical tradition. The pharmaceutical product, it is claimed, will *tame the psychotic fury.*

[13]Mancuso (1989) has offered the felicitous suggestion that we employ the descriptor *absurdity* to designate disvalued conduct.

been disappointing. The beliefs inherent in this world view guided scientists and practitioners to look upon human beings as organismic objects. From this perspective, it was assumed that the behavior of organisms could be understood, predicted, and controlled through applying the root metaphor of mechanistic science—the transmission of forces. From this belief there flowed countless hypotheses about the internal transmission and transformation of forces. Explanations of conduct, especially deviant conduct, focused on the transmission of forces within the brain.

The mechanistic world view is not the only metaphysical framework. An alternate framework, contextualism, leads to a totally different approach to the understanding of deviant conduct. The root metaphor of contextualism is the historical act in all its complexity. Change, novelty, variation, and contingency are the categories. Unlike mechanistic constructions in which the person is a passive object reacting to happenings within the body, the contextualist perspective directs the scientist to perceive human beings as agents, actors, and performers. Within this framework, the clinician would begin his study by posing questions such as "What is the person trying to do or say? What goals is he or she trying to reach? What story is he or she trying to tell?" Persons are perceived as agents trying—sometimes with shabby equipment—to maintain their self-narratives in the face of a complex, unpredictable, and confusing world. As agents, they may choose to incorporate into their sense-making the moral valuations imposed on their conduct by parents, siblings, employers, doctors, or other power figures. I see the failure of modern research on absurd conduct as following from the perception of "schizophrenics" as without agency, as suffering from happenings in the brain, rather than as agents trying to solve existential and identity problems through the construction of atypical beliefs, unusual imaginings, and nonconforming speech and gestural behavior. Were we to look upon such persons as agents we would become interested in how they arrive at constructions of the world that are so different from our own.

One implication of adopting a contextualist framework would be a reduction in the obsessive concern with diagnosis. Each person has his or her own story; the expressed beliefs, the atypical imaginings, the instrumental acts of withdrawing from strain-producing situations are intentional acts designed to solve identity and existential problems. The actions designed to keep one's self-narrative consistent are not invariant or machine-like outcomes of postulated disease processes. Contingencies of many kinds enter into the person's adopting a deviant role and also—I hasten to add—rejecting such a role.

Although current emphasis is on neuroscience, a respectable minority of professionals has been exploring methods for dealing with diagnosed schizophrenics as active participants in forming or changing their life narratives. The work of Strauss (1989), for example, departs radically from the prototypical neuroscience approach in that the patient is seen as a goal-directed being, as an agent. Understanding the patient's self-narrative is central to psychosocial therapeutic efforts (Sarbin, 1986). We can revive the case study which provides patients with the opportunity to reconstruct their self-narratives. Listening to patients' self-narratives is the first step in granting them the status of agents, of goal-directed beings. At the same time that patients reconstruct their life-narratives, they are given the opportunity of recounting the conduct of significant others who have collaborated in forming the self-narratives. To account for the themes in a self-narrative requires a vocabulary of relationships, rather than the usual language of individual pathology: toxins, tumors, trauma, complexes, dysfunctional traits, or defective genes.

It is instructive to note that the willingness to perceive the patient or client as agent has not been entirely obliterated by the popularity of "anti-psychotic" medication. In this connection, it is appropriate to raise the question of relative effectiveness of neuroleptic and psychosocial treatments. Karon (1989) reviewed the literature in which medication, placebo, and psychosocial interventions were compared; the studies employed a wide variety of criteria. The data are complex because of variations in experience of therapists, selection of schizophrenic patients, and dosages of medication. His overall conclusions, however, make clear that *in the long run* psychosocial treatments—in which the patient participates as an agent—have better outcomes than medications. The conclusions apply to such criteria as relapse rates, number of days in hospital, and relative costs.[14]

Schizophrenia: Diagnosis or Verdict?

In tracing the construction of schizophrenia, it becomes apparent that although masked as a medical diagnosis, schizophrenia is essentially

---

[14]Space limitations preclude a review of contributions by Estroff (1989), Goldstein (1987), Strauss (1989), Karon and VandenBos (1981), Wolkon and Peterson (1986), and others who have shown the value of psychosocial treatments, even though working within the schizophrenia or mental illness framework. The recognition of agency in such treatment programs is contradictory to the mechanistic view that regards behavioral acts as *happenings* and as the inevitable result of disease processes.

a moral verdict. The conduct that leads persons into the diagnosis-treatment sequence is initially the target of value judgments by others who have greater social power. The reports of these judgments accompany the putative patients when they enter the clinician's consulting room. The reports inform the diagnostician that certain actions of the pre-patients have not met the normative standards of others. This bare fact is the starting point for the whole schizophrenia enterprise: conduct exhibited by one person is assigned a negative moral judgment by another. Since normative standards against which conduct is judged are contingent on time, place, and person, the notion of a universal disease process is irrelevant and misleading.

Employing a different vocabulary, Trigant Burrow, eminent psychiatrist, psychoanalyst, social critic, and author, anticipated in the 1920s the idea of the social construction of schizophrenia when he wrote:

> Of dementia praecox, the disease, psychiatry is in fact more a cause than a cure, just as mothers and doctors who habitually hold to a mental attitude of personal ministration and concern...are more an occasion than a remedy for disease in general. And so the real disorder, after all, is not dementia praecox but psychiatry. When the psychiatrist will have come to understand dementia praecox,...this objective figment of his own disordered consciousness will spontaneously vanish (Burrow, 1927, p. 137).

References

Abrams, R. & Taylor, M.A. (1983). The genetics of schizophrenia: A reassessment using modern criteria. *American Journal of Psychiatry*, 140, 171-175.

Andreasen, N.C. (1982). Negative symptoms in schizophrenia: Definition and reliability. *Archives of General Psychiatry*, 39, 784-788.

Bateson, G., Jackson, D.D., Haley, J., & Weakland, J.H. (1956). Toward a theory of schizophrenia. *Behavioral Science*, 1, 251-264.

Benjamin, L.S. (1976). A reconsideration of the Kety and Associates study of genetic factors in the transmission of schizophrenia. *American Journal of Psychiatry*, 133, 1129-1133.

Benjamin, L.S. (1989). Is chronicity a function of the relationship between the person and auditory hallucination? *Schizophrenia Bulletin*, 15, 291-310.

Bentall, R.P., Jackson, H.F., & Pilgrim, D. (1988). Abandoning the concept of 'schizophrenia:' Some implications of validity arguments for psychological research into psychotic phenomena. *British Journal of Clinical Psychology*, 27, 303-324.

Blashfield, R.K., Sprock, J., & Fuller, A.K. (1990). Suggested guidelines for including or excluding categories in the DSM-IV. *Comprehensive Psychiatry*, 31, 15-19.

Blum, J.D. (1978). On changes in psychiatric diagnosis over time. *American Psychologist*, 33, 1017-1031.

Boyle, M. (1990). Is schizophrenia what it was? A reanalysis of Kraepelin's and Bleuler's population. *Journal of the History of the Behavioral Sciences*, (in press).

Breggin, P.R. (1983). *Psychiatric drugs: Hazards to the brain.* New York: Springer.

Broen, W.C. & Nakamura, C. (1972). Reduced range of sensory sensitivity in chronic nonparanoid schizophrenics. *Journal of Abnormal Psychology, 79,* 106-111.

Burrow, T. (1927). *The social basis of consciousness.* New York: Harcourt Brace & Co.

Carpenter, W.T., Jr., & Kirkpatrick, B. (1988). The heterogeneity of the long term course of schizophrenia. *Schizophrenia Bulletin, 14,* 645-652.

Cohen, D. (1989). Biological basis of schizophrenia: The evidence reconsidered. *Social Work, 34,* 247-257.

Cohen, D. & Cohen, H. (1986). Biological theories, drug treatments, and schizophrenia: A critical assessment. *Journal of Mind and Behavior, 7,* 11-35.

Clementz, B.A. & Sweeney, J.A. (1990). Is eye movement dysfunction a biological marker for schizophrenia? A methodological review. *Psychological Bulletin, 108,* 77-92.

Craik, K.H. (1959). The Cosans versus the Cnidians, or comments on diagnosis in general and diagnosis of schizophrenia in particular. Berkeley: University of California (unpublished manuscript).

Dohrenwend, B.P. (1990). Socioeconomic status (SES) and psychiatric disorders: Are the issues still compelling? *Social Psychiatry and Psychiatric Epidemiology, 25,* 41-47.

Ellard, J. (1987). Did schizophrenia exist before the eighteenth century? *Australian and New Zealand Journal of Psychiatry, 21,* 306-314.

Estroff, S.E. (1989). Self, identity, and subjective experiences of schizophrenia: In search of the subject. *Schizophrenia Bulletin, 15,* 189-195.

Goldstein, M.J. (1987). Psychosocial issues. *Schizophrenia Bulletin, 13,* 157-171.

Gottesman, J.J. & Shields, J. (1972). *Schizophrenia and genetics.* New York: Academic Press.

Gubrium, J. & Holstein, J.A. (1990). *What is family?* Mountainview, CA: Mayfield Publishing Co.

Hays, P. (1984). The nosological status of schizophrenia. *Lancet,* 1342-1345.

Hoffer, A. & Mahon, M. (1961). The presence of unidentified substances in the urine of schizophrenic patients. *Journal of Neuropsychiatry, 2,* 331-362.

Hoffer, A. & Osmund, H. (1963). Malvaria: A new psychiatric disease. *Acta Psychiatrica Scandinavia, 39,* 355-366.

Juhasz, J.B. & Sarbin, T.R. (1966). On the false alarm metaphor in psychophysics. *Psychological Record, 16,* 323-327.

Karon, B. P. (1989). Psychotherapy versus medication for schizophrenia: Empirical considerations. In Fisher, S. & Greenberg, R.P. (Eds.), *The limits of biological treatments for psychological stress.,* Hillsdale, NJ: Lawrence Erlbaum Associates.

Karon, B.P. & VandenBos, G.R. (1981). *Psychotherapy of schizophrenia: The treatment of choice.* New York: Aronson.

Kety, S.S. (1974). From rationalization to reason. *American Journal of Psychiatry, 103,* 957-962.

Kety, S.S., Rosenthal, D., Wender, P.H., & Shulsinger, P. (1968). The types and prevalence of mental illness in the biological and adoptive families of adoptive schizophrenics. In Rosenthal, D. & Kety, S.S. (Eds.), *The transmission of schizophrenia.* New York: Pergamon.

Kety, S.S., Rosenthal, D., Wender, P.H., Shulsinger, F., & Jacobson, B. (1975). Mental illness in the biological and adoptive families of adoptive individuals who have become schizophrenic: A preliminary report based upon psychiatric interviews. In Fieve, R., Rosenthal, D., & Brill, H. (Eds.) *Genetic research in psychiatry.* Baltimore: Johns Hopkins Press.

Kraepelin, E. (1908). *Lectures on clinical psychiatry.* New York: Hafner.

Kringlen, E. & Cramer, G. (1989). Offspring of monozygotic twins discordant for schizophrenia. *Archives of General Psychiatry, 46,* 873-877.

Landrine, H. (1989). The social class-schizophrenia relationship: A different approach and new hypotheses. *Social and Clinical Psychology, 8,* 288-303.

Lewontin, R.C., Kamin, L., & Rose, S. (1984). *Not in our genes: Biology, ideology, and human nature.* New York: Pantheon.

Lidz, T. (1990). Optimism in treatment of schizophrenia still premature, says expert. *Psychiatric News, 25,* 26-33.

Lidz, T. & Blatt, S. (1983). Critiques of Danish-American studies of biological and adoptive relatives of adoptees who became schizophrenic. *American Journal of Psychiatry, 140,* 426-435.

Lidz, T., Blatt, S., & Cook, B. (1981). Critique of Danish-American studies of adopted-away offspring of schizophrenic parents. *American Journal of Psychiatry, 138,* 1063-1068.

Loranger, A.W. (1990). The impact of DSM-III on diagnostic practice in a university hospital: A comparison of DSM-II and DSM-III on 10,914 patients. *Archives of General Psychiatry, 47,* 672-675.

Mancuso, J.C. (1989). Review of Porter, R. *A social history of madness: The world through the eyes of the insane.* New York: Weidenfeld and Nicolson, 1988. In *Society, July-August,* 92-94.

Marshall, R. (1986). Hereditary aspects of schizophrenia: A critique. In Eisenberg, N. & Glasgow, D. (Eds.) *Current issues in clinical psychology.* Brookfield, VT: Gower.

Meehl, P. (1989). Schizotaxia revisited. *Archives of General Psychiatry, 46,* 935-944.

Mesulam, M.M. (1990). Schizophrenia and the brain. *New England Journal of Medicine, 322,* 842-845.

Pavkov, T.W., Lewis, D.A., & Lyons, J.S. (1989). Diagnosis and racial bias: An empirical investigation. *Professional Psychology, Research and Practice, 20,* 384-368.

Raz, S. & Raz, N. (1990). Structural brain abnormalities in the major psychoses: A quantitative review of evidence from computerized imaging. *Psychological Bulletin, 108,* 93-108.

Rosenberg, C.E. (1989). Disease in history: Frames and framers. *Milbank Quarterly, 67,* Supplement 1, 1-15.

Rosenhan, D. (1973). On being sane in insane places. *Science, 179,* 250-258.

Sarbin, T.R. (1967). The concept of hallucination. *Journal of Personality, 35,* 359-380.

Sarbin, T.R. (1969). Schizophrenic thinking: A role-theory interpretation. *Journal of Personality, 37,* 190-206.

Sarbin, T.R. (1972a). Imagining as muted role-taking: A historico-linguistic analysis. In Sheehan, P. (Ed.), *The function and nature of imagery.* New York: Academic Press.

Sarbin, T.R. (1972b). Schizophrenia: From metaphor to myth. *Psychology Today, June,* 1972.

Sarbin, T.R. (1986). *Narrative psychology: The storied nature of human conduct.* New York: Praeger.

Sarbin, T.R. (1990). Metaphors of unwanted conduct: A historical sketch. In Leary, D. (Ed.), *The history of metaphor in psychology.* New York: Cambridge University Press.

Sarbin, T.R. & Juhasz, J.B. (1967). The historical background of the concept of hallucination. *Journal of the History of the Behavioral Sciences, 3,* 339-358.

Sarbin, T.R. & Juhasz, J.B. (1970). Toward a theory of imagination. *Journal of Personality, 38,* 52-76.

Sarbin, T.R. & Juhasz, J.B. (1975). The social psychology of hallucination. In Siegel, R. & West, L.J. (Eds.) *Hallucination: Theory and research.* New York: Wiley.

Sarbin, T.R. & Juhasz, J.B. (1978). The social psychology of hallucinations. *Journal of Mental Imagery, 2,* 117-144.

Sarbin, T.R. & Juhasz, J.B. (1982). The concept of mental illness: A historical perspective. In Al-Issa, I. (Ed.) *Culture and psychopathology*. Baltimore: University Park Press.

Sarbin, T.R. & Mancuso, J.C. (1980). *Schizophrenia: Medical diagnosis or moral verdict?* Elmsford, NY: Pergamon Press.

Sarbin, T.R., Mancuso, J.C., & Podczerwinski, J. (in preparation). A critical review of research on schizophrenia reported in the *Journal of Abnormal Psychology*, 1959-1988.

Schneider, K. (1959). *Clinical psychopathology*. New York: Grune and Stratton.

Scull, A. (1987). Desperate remedies: A Gothic tale of madness and modern medicine. *Psychological Medicine, 17*, 561-577.

Siegler, M. & Osmund, H. (1973). Aesculapian authority. *Hastings Center Studies, 1*, 41-52.

Singer, M.T. & Wynne, L.C. (1963). Differentiating characteristics of the parents of childhood neurotics and young adult schizophrenics. *American Journal of Psychiatry, 120*, 234-243.

Strauss, J.S. (1989). Subjective experiences of schizophrenia: Toward a new dynamic psychiatry—II. *Schizophrenia Bulletin, 15*, 179-187.

Thornton, C. & Gottheil, E. (1971). Social schemata in schizophrenic males. *Journal of Abnormal Psychology, 77*, 192-195.

Valenstein, E.S. (1986). *Great and desperate cures: The rise and decline of psychosurgery and other radical treatments for mental illness*. New York: Basic Books.

van den Brink, W., Koeter, M.W.J., Ormel, J., Dijkstra, W., Giel, R., Sloof, C.J., & Woolfarth, T.D. (1989). Psychiatric diagnosis in an outpatient population: A comparative study of PSE-Catego and DSM-III. *Archives of General Psychiatry, 46*, 369-372.

Warner, R. (1985). *Recovery from schizophrenia: Psychiatry and political economy*. Boston: Routledge & Kegan Paul.

Wing, J., Cooper, J., & Sartorius, N. (1974). *The description and classification of psychiatric symptoms: An instruction manual for PSE and Catego system*. London: Cambridge University Press.

White, H. (1972). The forms of wildness: Archeology of an idea. In Dudley, E. & Novick, M.E. (Eds.) , *The wild man within*. Pittsburgh: University of Pittsburgh Press.

Wolkon, G.H., & Peterson, C.L. (1986). A conceptual framework for the psychosocial rehabilitation of the chronic mental patient. *Psychosocial Rehabilitation Journal, 9*, 43-55.

14
Schizophrenia: A Defective, Deficient, Disrupted, Disorganized Construct
Morton Wiener

Terms such as psychopathology, deviancy, psychosis, schizophrenia, and their subsets, are part of a traditional paradigm in which some unusual instances of psychosocial actions are tc be understood, described, and explained. In this tradition, behaviors that are deemed unacceptable or disruptive for a socio-cultural group are said to be explained by, caused by, or attributable to some defect, deficiency, disruption, or disorganization of some agency *within* the person (i.e., distorted cognitions, genes, attention deficit, enlarged ventricle, etc.). Such explanation seems nothing more than a technological variant of the historical invocation of "possession". A corollary belief in this tradition is that a different explanation is required for such unusual events than is required for other unusual events (e.g., bravery, altruism), or for the usual, typical, and familiar kinds of psychosocial actions. Three interrelated issues are quickly apparent. There are questions about the coherence of the underlying metaphor in this tradition; about the presumption of distinctive differences between the behaviors considered abnormal and those behaviors considered normative; and about many contradictions and problems evident in the empirical efforts to investigate "schizophrenia". The issues and arguments raised here about this tradition in general, and schizophrenia specifically, are similar to those raised in an analysis of depression (Wiener, 1989) and of anorexia nervosa (Marcus & Wiener, 1989).

In contrast to the traditional view of internal causation and a discontinuity between the psychosocial action patterns now considered disordered or deviant, and those considered typical, usual, or normative, the argument is that (1) the ostensibly atypical patterns of psychosocial actions are clearly analogous to other psychosocial actions that are considered normal, or even desirable; (2) there is a specifiable continuity of the so-called unusual and usual behaviors, including their bio-physio-chemical substrates (i.e., correlates) over the populations at large; (3) differences between individuals in psychosocial transactions can be compared and contrasted in the same ways we consider, compare, or contrast sub-cultural, ethnic, or cultural groups; and (4) these identified behavioral patterns can be explained (or accounted for) by the same sets of terms we invoke to account for the more usual or typical instances of psychosocial actions. If it can be shown that the psychosocial events that have been considered strange or unique in the traditional perspectives (the bases for identifying the individuals of interest) are frequent and considered normative for some socio-cultural group or subgroup, then the traditional belief that these kinds of psychosocial actions must be pathological, or signs of pathologies *in the person* may no longer be considered reasonable. Further, if the equivalence of typical actions and those unusual (schizophrenic) psychosocial actions can be demonstrated, this demonstration would argue against the use of category terms that connote defect, deficiency, disruption, or disorganization in the person to explain these kind of socio-culturally designated instances.

Arguments for a paradigm that is different from one that has prevailed for a considerable time and has become part of the everyday language of a socio-cultural group, seem to require a different kind of logic and coherence than those that are required to emend a traditional perspective. To question the coherence of such constructs as psychopathology, psychosis, deviancy, and schizophrenia and to suggest a different paradigm, requires arguments that not only deal with issues, but must also anticipate the incredulity of traditionalists.

Paradigms and Metaphors

Kuhn (1972) claimed that new paradigms—that is, changes from one set of assumptions, categories, and inferences to another—are attempts to incorporate some of the imprecision, ambiguities, contradictions, and overgeneralizations that are overlooked or ignored, often *on pragmatic grounds*, by investigators working within the traditional paradigm of an era. Further, Kuhn makes the claim that an alternative paradigm need be no less scientific than the traditional view. The difference between the traditional and the newer paradigm is that objects (or events) grouped in one way in the traditional view are grouped differently in the new paradigm. When asked to clarify the concept of "paradigm" in his usage, Kuhn described it as a "disciplinary matrix," a most interesting play on words that connotes both the discourse of a discipline and its coercive quality.

Turbayne (1970), in a similar endeavor, noted the seductiveness of a "metaphor" and the "loss of the metaphor" in description and explanation. He notes that in his usage, metaphor encompasses all kinds of "cross-sorting"; in the same way, Ryle (1949) uses "category error." Turbayne also cites Black's (1954) claim that in some cases the metaphor *creates* the similarity rather than being taken from some existing similarity. Further, *metaphor*, taken as the presentation of the facts of one category in the idioms appropriate to another, is not constrained to language, but can readily be expanded to include other representations (e.g., models, diagrams). Turbayne claimed that with common usage of terms (terms that are metaphors) in descriptions and explanations, the "as if" changes to "is." With this transformation, an epistemological proposition very soon attains ontological status.

The basic debate, then, in arguments about perspectives, is *not* about facts per se, but about premises and categories. That is, what kinds of observations, by what kinds of observers, with what kinds of operations, categories, and measurements, are deemed appropriate or relevant for a particular paradigm or metaphor. To the extent that pragmatic grounds are often a fundamental justification for maintaining a traditional perspective, it is important to note that all paradigms include pragmatic consequences, but that a different perspective may entail different consequences than those deemed appropriate in a traditional approach (i.e., institutionalization, psychotherapy, lobotomy, medication, etc.).

Raising doubts about the prevailing traditional paradigm may be less daunting if one remembers that whenever a traditional metaphor has been questioned, it has not been unusual to find heated dismissals of the criticisms until an alternative becomes the traditional metaphor. In the history of psychology and psychiatry, many traditions have given way to newer ones; and in each era, investigators believed that their current perspective was the only reasonable formulation.

The first issue of concern here, is that a special kind of explanation has become a prerequisite for those unusual psychosocial actions that are now labeled as psychopathological, but not for other analogous unusual psychosocial actions. It is quite evident that different socio-cultural groups identify different kinds of events as unusual. Some events are considered disruptive for the group and may even call forth social sanctions (e.g., "crimes"), while others are deemed facilitating for the group and are lauded (e.g., heroism, altruism). However, the rationale for invoking different sorts of "agency" (i.e., defect, deficiency, disruption, or disorganization) for those events considered socially disruptive, but not for those unusual events considered facilitating by a socio-cultural group is unclear. The issue here is not what kinds of actions or events are identified; rather, it is about the particular explanatory principles that are invoked for particular subsets of atypical psychosocial transactions—in this case, schizophrenia, which is considered disruptive for the group.

Before we explore the traditional explanations, it is important to note some apparent inconsistencies in the traditional metaphor of psychopathology. For example, those investigators who hold a social construction view of schizophrenia consider the unusual psychosocial *action* to be defective, deficient, disrupted, disorganized, and therefore the "pathology." Others (e.g., those in the medical-disease perspective) view these psychosocial actions as only a *sign* or symptom of some internal isomorphic defect, deficiency, disruption, or disorganization. In the latter case, the as yet unidentified, internal event is the pathology. All too often, the sign and the internal event are considered isomorphic. If one accepts the sign-symptom perspective, what are the grounds for grouping the individual on the bases of ostensible commonality of *behavioral* actions without evidence of a one-to-one correspondence of these variable psychosocial behaviors with a *specific*, common substrate—one that has not yet been identified despite almost one hundred years of effort.

Traditional Paradigm

There has also been a continuing effort to maintain the traditional paradigm by recategorizing and sub-categorizing schizophrenia. Such efforts are clearly evident in the successive editions of the *Diagnostic and Statistical Manual of Mental Disorders*. The changes in each succeeding edition can be interpreted as ways to incorporate some of the apparent ambiguity and impreciseness found in earlier efforts to categorize the many different psychosocial action patterns subsumed under schizophrenia. (One can also view the efforts to establish a diagnostic and statistical manual as an attempt to codify the traditional paradigm, that is, to establish a "disciplinary matrix," in both senses of this term.) Although the newly created sub-categories may be necessary to eliminate some ambiguities or discrepancies, the new distinctions are considered to be only refinements of the previous non-differentiated categories. The individuals in each of the newly created sub-categories (e.g., Hebephrenic types or Acute Schizophrenia episode) are assumed to still share some commonality with the individuals in all of the other sub-categories (e.g., Catatonic type or Residual type): each of the individuals was a member of a homogeneous group, the earlier undifferentiated precursor category (i.e., Schizophrenia). Significant differences in the psychosocial transactions of individuals within a classification are also ignored. (See Marcus & Wiener, 1989, for an example of such differences for the diagnosis "anorexia," and Wiener, 1989, for "depression".) Unfortunately, besides tradition, the grounds for maintaining a unity among the sub-categories (e.g., catatonic, schizoaffective, paranoid type, "schizophrenic disorders" or even maintaining that individuals diagnosed as "delusional" and socially isolated, can be grouped with those considered delusional and socially intrusive) are less than obvious. What, other than tradition, do these categories have in common if it is not the commonalities of psychosocial actions or a biochemical or physiological substrate that has yet to be identified?

Once it becomes evident that the behavioral diversity is too great to reconcile, the arguments move to "formal" similarity; that is, an appeal to "diagnosis" as this term is understood in the medical tradition. Three perspectives can be identified in this continuing controversy. Shall, or shall we not consider "diagnoses" and medical-disease "pathology" as the way to understand schizophrenia. The arguments and data offered by the proponents of different perspectives—even for some who argue for a socio-cultural explanation—can be used to exemplify how the underlying metaphor is extended and reinterpreted. These reinterpretations maintain our traditional belief and metaphor that unusual or atypical actions are, or must continue to be viewed as, reflecting some defect, deficiency, disruption, or disorganization of the person.

The elaboration and reformulation of the traditional metaphor can be seen most clearly in what is now explicitly labeled the "medical-disease" model. When questions were raised about the coherence of the construct "mental illness" and of "disease" itself, investigators in this tradition redefined and extended the sense of these constructs. (See Kerr & Snaith [1986]; Spaulding & Cole [1984]). The further claim was made that any problem that may be modified by some physio-bio-chemical substance must be a disease. When further questions were raised about these extensions and their relevance for psychosocial actions incorporated under the concept of disease, the claim was made that even if no tissue dysfunction could be identified, these events (i.e., psychopathological psychosocial actions) still belong to medicine *because of tradition and pragmatic consequences.*

It is interesting to note the diversity of arguments and justifications invoked by the many investigators involved in the endeavors to maintain the traditional medical-disease paradigm for psycho-pathologies (e.g., American Psychiatric Association, 1987; Cloninger, Martin, Guze, & Clayton, 1985; Goodwin & Guze, 1984; Guze, 1970;

Kendell, 1975; 1986; Woodruff, Goodwin, & Guze, 1974). They argue that those questioning the traditional metaphor misunderstand the interrelated set of concepts—symptom, syndrome, diagnosis, disorder, mental illness and/or disease (e.g., Cloninger, Martin, Guze, & Clayton, 1985). Guze (in Woodruff, Goodwin & Guze, 1974) had claimed that:

> Classification has two functions: communication and prediction. Classification in medicine is called diagnosis... Diagnostic categories—diseases, illnesses, syndromes—are included if they have been sufficiently studied to be useful. Like roses a disease is a cluster of symptoms and/or signs with a *more or less* predictable course... *But whatever the psychiatric problems are, they have this in common with "real" diseases—they result in consultation with a physician and are associated with pain, suffering, disability, and death* (Preface VIII-IX, *emphasis* added).

Note that the metaphor is maintained by including "pain," "suffering," and "disability" (a "loss of the metaphor" in the sense of Turbayne, 1970), and by explicitly claiming the *usefulness* of the paradigm. Does discomfort or disruption of any kind (e.g., being lost in an unknown city) constitute pain and suffering in a medical sense, and is it therefore a disease? Incidently, Guze also offers the explicit argument that the traditional paradigm is accepted by the social community, with the inference that acceptance connotes validity. For Cloninger et al. (1985), the constructs of symptom, syndrome, diagnosis, disorder, and mental illness are considered to be facts; reliable classification is the only requirement. The underlying assumption appears to be that if one can show "reliable" classification (i.e., everyone includes the same kinds of instances into a category), then there *must* be some commonality among the members of a category. How does one distinguish classification consistent with a conceptual model versus conformity to socio-cultural constraints (e.g., going to church on Sunday in a small community).

Kendell (1982) invoked a somewhat different argument to maintain the medical disease metaphor:

> What are we really trying to do when we decide to identify a subgroup of *patients* as "schizophrenics" or "melancholics?" I suggest that, as practicing clinicians, we are usually trying to demarcate a group of patients with either a relatively homogeneous *treatment* response or a relatively homogeneous long-term outcome. As research

workers, however, we are probably trying to identify a group of patients whose *symptoms* have a common etiology or pathogenesis or who share an as yet *unidentified biological predisposition* (p. 1335, *emphasis* added).

Note here the identification of individuals as "patients," of "symptoms," and of individuals who receive "treatment," even though there is an explicit acknowledgment that there is no evidence of any known biological component that warrants a category of "patienthood."

More recently, Kendell (1986), acknowledged that despite the absence of reliable or consistent evidence of pathophysiology, or of genetic-biologic disadvantage factors to account for these kinds of unusual actions, as long as physicians and laymen agree that the ostensible dysfunction is a disease or a medical problem, then it is pragmatically useful to maintain the medical perspective. Kendell continued this kind of argument when he wrote, "By all means let us *insist* that schizophrenia is an illness and that we (psychiatrists) are better equipped to understand and treat it than anyone else" (p. 30).

What is also unclear when a disease metaphor is invoked is whether the "disease" is to be considered to be similar to pneumonia, a broken leg, or childbirth (which must be seen as a disease since physicians "treat" them; they are traditional; and each involves "pain" and "suffering") or to Down's syndrome, multiple sclerosis, Huntington's chorea, or sickle-cell anemia. When investigators write about most psychopathologies including depression, the term "disease" seems to be used as if it belongs in the first group, but when the concept is applied to schizophrenia or manic depression, it seems to be used in ways that would incorporate it in the second group. That is, we can "cure" the former, but we can only keep the latter under some kind of "control" by our interventions. As far as can be determined in the claims cited above, tradition and convention are the rationales for maintaining the paradigm and its metaphor. After almost one hundred years of effort, data have yet to be uncovered that demonstrate any common defect, deficiency, disruption, or disorganization among those individuals identified as schizophrenic or as members of any of its subsets; nor is there evidence that the purported treatment has anything to do with the purported defects, deficiencies, disruptions, or disorganization.

Sign, Symptom, Classification, and Stereotype

Let us turn to the construct diagnosis and the concepts of *signs* and *symptoms*. "Sign" is taken to be an observable event, "symptoms" as self-reports about events not otherwise available to an observer. Diagnosis, signs, and symptoms connote that there is something more than, or even other than, the constellation of psychosocial actions that are used to assign the label. This kind of usage is clearly a different sort of classification than the categorization of someone as a lawyer, poet, or physician. It is unclear, then, whether diagnosis is to be understood only as a classification (e.g., lawyer, poet, or physician), a prototypical description, a stereotype, or a term clearly connoting something else (e.g., some internal bio-physio-chemical dysfunction).

If diagnosis is only a conventional term, and means nothing more than "classification," then it is important to acknowledge explicitly that the psychosocial actions are the "psychopathology," and that is a social-cultural convention. This conclusion is congruent with those drawn by others in some recent literature reviews of classification (e.g., Baker, 1986; Rosch, 1978; Smith, Balzano, & Walker, 1978; Smith & Medin, 1981; Smith, Shobin, & Rips, 1974). One focal question raised in all of this literature is whether the bases for classification are attributes (i.e., features) of the objects, or imposed social conventions. For example, what criteria constitute the category of "tools" (does it include razor blade or strop), or of "furniture" (does it include "toilet seat") as opposed to the criteria for a category like "butterfly?" If a diagnosis of schizophrenia is to be understood as a classification, (with disjunctive criteria including onset, duration of symptoms, age of the person, and cultural context), is it a classification more like "tool" or "furniture" than like "rose" or "bird" (categories which are ostensibly designated by morphological or other biological criteria)?

Some investigators (e.g., Cantor, Smith, French-deSales, & Mezzick, 1980) argue that the concept "prototypicality" can deal with the diversity of symptoms and signs in diagnosis, and that the diversity of appearances need not be of concern. Their argument seems to be that diversity of appearances occurs in all classification, and that "features" (i.e., criterial attributes) need only be *correlated* with group membership. A prototype, then, is the item(s) that *judges* consider the best exemplar(s) of a class. That is, the more agreement there is about an instance as an exemplar, the more prototypical it is. When there is less agreement among the judges, such instances are only considered less prototypical. Unfortunately, the examples used to argue for this approach usually includes categories such as "birds" rather than "tools." When "tools" are scaled for prototype, the scale is ordered by familiarity and common use rather than by features. Such findings appear to be examples of social convention, not inherent commonality. A further assumption in a prototypical scale approach (similar to that of Cloninger et al., 1985) is that if a scale of prototypicality can be generated, there must be some underlying commonality. However, as Wiener (1989) noted, one could as easily develop a prototype of dragons, gods, or aliens from outer space, as one could for the category of "schizophrenics." If prototypicality only represents social convention, then it does not seem to be a reasonable argument for presumed commonality. As noted earlier, one can readily interpret the prototypical criteria specified in the Diagnostic and Statistical Manuals as dicta to *impose* consensuality (a disciplinary matrix). No evidence has yet been offered that consensuality (i.e., reliable diagnosis) arises from the instances to be judged.

Unfortunately, socio-cultural categorizations of individuals more often than not evolve into stereotypes rather than remaining a classification, or even a prototype. Once a categorization becomes a stereotype, then anyone with any of the features is deemed to have the other attributes as well, latently or incipiently. Unfortunately, there is also some empirical evidence in the social psychology literature that once a group of individuals are labeled, the label itself becomes the basis for a stereotype. That is, users seem to note ostensible similarities among the individuals assigned the label; any differences between individuals in this category are ignored, any similarities between members and non-members of the category are similarly ignored. This kind of socio-cultural transformation has been demonstrated by Tajfel and his colleagues. Tajfel, et al., (1963; 1964; 1978) explored the social consequences of arbitrarily assigning "normal" individuals, randomly selected from the general population, to an arbitrarily labeled group. That is, randomly selected individuals were labeled as belonging to a "J" group. Despite the random selection of subjects from the *same* larger group, and an arbitrary label assigned to the group, judges, when asked to view this J group, proceeded to identify common attributes for these individuals that they claimed were not evident for these individuals who were not in the randomly selected group.

One can infer, then, that labeling of individuals as belonging to a group engenders a belief that the members must share some significant commonality; that is, a labeling of individuals engenders stereotyping. Scheff (1966; 1974) offered a similar argument about "labeling."

Further, the more strongly a stereotype is held, the more there is a presumption that there is a high degree of similarity (if not identity) among group members, as well as a belief that clear-cut differences exist between the stereotyped group and other individuals. On the other hand, the more one has contact with members of a group, the greater the awareness of the many differences among group members, and the similarity of these members to non-stereotyped individuals. If a diagnostic category (e.g., psychopathology) is a stereotype or a label, we would not be surprised to find that clinicians and other investigators respond the same way as subjects do in social psychology studies.

Nonexclusiveness of Signs and Symptom

One way to raise doubts about a "diagnosis" approach, in general, and the construct of "schizophrenia" in particular, is to try to show that the signs and symptoms taken to be criterial for schizophrenia are also evident in the general population. "Positive" signs and symptoms (i.e., hallucination, delusion, thought disorder) and "negative" signs and symptoms (i.e., alogia, flattened affect, anhedonia, asociality, attentional impairment, and apathy) are often considered as criteria for labeling someone as schizophrenic.

The argument to be made here is that the same signs or symptoms can be found for individuals who are not considered schizophrenic. The clearest example is in the explicit caveat in DSM-III-R that individuals in some contexts who manifest signs or symptoms are *not* to be considered pathological.

> When an experience or behavior is entirely normative for a particular culture—e.g., the experience of hallucinating the voice of the deceased in the first few weeks of bereavement in various North American Indian groups, or trance and possession states occurring in culturally approved ritual contexts in much of the non-Western world—it should not be regarded as pathological. Culture-specific symptoms of distress, such as particular somatic symptoms associated with distress in members of different ethnic and cultural groups may create difficulties in the use of DSM-III-R, because the *psychopathology* is unique to that culture or because the DSM-III-R categories are

not based on extensive research with non-Western populations.[1] (Preface XXVI; *emphasis* added)

Two points are particularly cogent in this DSM-III-R caveat. One is the acknowledgment that reports of distress are part of the language, values, behavioral norms, and idiomatic expressions of a culture. The other is that the very same actions we consider clear-cut evidence of schizophrenia (that is, hallucinations, trance, and possession states) are not to be considered "pathological" *if they are part of a cultural belief.* From such assertions, it is clear then that such psychosocial events are not pathological in themselves. If it is not the act, what is the pathology? It seems reasonable to infer that different beliefs may be held by different ethnic or other sub-groups within the larger community about some "unusual events" (e.g., "Obeah" in some Caribbean communities), or by other subsets of individuals (e.g., religious denominations, including God-seekers). Is it not also reasonable to consider every report we consider an hallucination (not attributable to toxic conditions) as representing a difference in language, socio-cultural values, behavioral or idiomatic expressions, rather than pathology?

Further, Sarbin (1967, and in this volume), among others, has argued that hallucinations are not in themselves unusual in the general population, nor are they particularly disturbing to the person reporting them, or to a person listening to these reports in certain contexts (e.g., therapy). We would not find reports of hallucinations disturbing in autobiographical reports from people we "respect," or in certain contexts (intense emotion-invoking instances), or in particular eras (e.g., the time of Joan of Arc or the time of Jesus Christ). Shall we infer that someone is schizophrenic if that person were to report, "Whenever I go home, I still see my father sitting in his favorite chair," or "I saw a UFO," or "Jesus came to me...," or "I hear God's voice telling me to stop abortions," or "I felt myself incorporated and I became my mother at that moment"? How would we evaluate individuals we consider "God-seekers," or who report "trance" states and similar unusual experiences? Are these different *kinds* of hallucinations, or do we judge them as metaphorical "as if" claims, or as "unfounded" interpretations of indistinct, ambiguous stimuli viewed under emotionally charged contexts? In what ways are these different

---

[1]This text is contradictory when the clause such as "because the psychopathology is unique to that culture..." is added. How can something be considered both normative for a population and "pathological"?

than the kinds of reports we hear from individuals labeled schizophrenic?

As for "delusions," there is the often quoted statement, "My beliefs and claims are real and reasonable; yours are delusions." There are a number of issues surrounding the concept of delusion. One obvious problem is, who is to decide what is to be considered possible or reasonable for whom? For example, what are we to make about claims that life as we know it occurs in other galaxies; or that there are plots against a particular ethnic or sub-cultural group; or that the CIA plotted and carried out the assassination of President Kennedy; or that "I wasn't hired because of my religion or skin color." Shall we consider it "delusional" if an "African-American" claims that "whites are out to destroy us," or a "Caucasian" claims that "Blacks want to destroy us by miscegenation." It is not clear what grounds are to be used to decide that there must be something "wrong" with someone when he or she believes something other than what most people believe are the "facts." Although some of these "unusual" interpretations may be socially *unacceptable* or disagreeable, disagreement with, or non-congruence, with societal norms does not seem to warrant the term "pathological." More often than not, the term "delusion" seems to be applied when someone offers a non-consensual interpretation, or when the content can be said to be socially *intrusive*.

When a statement or claim is labeled a delusion, there is a correlated inference that the person who is making that statement or claim must be "disordered." There are, on the other hand, examples of non-consensual claims, explanations or attributions about events that are considered to be "appropriate," "a revelation," or "creative." How is one to decide if a claim that "we must destroy the communist menace" is a socio-political "truth" or a delusion? What are we to make of claims made by Jehovah's Witnesses about the imminent destruction of the earth; claims made by those who believe in reincarnation, or statements that abortionists are performing the work of the Devil? What about claims that the world will be destroyed by changes in the ozone layers, or by other environmental "pollutants." Are these any different than "I have plans for an extremely high efficiency engine that the industrialists want to destroy," or "There have been numerous sightings of UFOs, but the government is suppressing these facts."? Are the followers of Reverend Moon, or of a guru, or those who established a colony in Jonestown, to be considered deficient, defective, disruptive, or disorganized; but at the same time are others who held out a similar possibility for an utopian society (e.g., Bellamy, Skinner, Thoreau) to be considered socio-culturally imaginative?

If we now look to the negative signs, that is, behaviors that do not occur (more aptly described as social actions that are not like those of the "majority"), we find a clear socio-economic class correlation. Landrine (1989), concerned about this ostensible relationship of schizophrenia and social class—particularly relationship of the negative symptoms to a diagnosis of schizophrenia—details the extensive overlap of the language patterns of "schizophrenics" and the language and cultural patterns of the "working class" or "underclass" individuals in America. She also reported how easy it was for clinicians to "diagnose" *stereotypical* examples of lower class speech as meeting the criteria of "schizophrenia" or of a "schizotypal personality." Landrine quotes segments of a paper by Schatzman and Strauss (1955). These authors had noted that:

> ... (our) sample of normal poor subjects spoke in "dream-like sets of images with few connective, qualifying, explanatory, or other context-providing devices" and were "likely to wander off into detail about a particular incident ... Often one incident becomes the trigger for another, and although some logical or temporal connection between them may exist for the speaker, this can scarcely be perceived by the interviewer. The great danger of probes and requests for elaboration is that the speaker will get far away from the lifeline of his narrative—and frequently far away from the interviewer's question. [We found that] [g]eneral questions are especially likely to divert the speaker, since they suggest only loose frames; or he may answer in general, diffuse, or blurred terms ... [T]he respondent may ... completely reconstruct incidents that seem only partially connected with each other or with his narrative ... Some literally cannot tell a straight story or describe a simple incident coherently. At the other extreme we find an adequate self-focused narrative, with considerable detail tightly tied to sequential action, including retrospective observation about the narrator's facts as he develops them. Midway between these ... are people who can tell portions of narrative, but are easily distracted (quoted verbatim from Landrine, 1989, pp. 293-294).

The point here is not to describe social class differences in communication, but rather to point out that although we consider certain *forms of behavior* pathological (and presume that they require special explanation), we can also find the very same kinds of occurrences when we explore the communication behaviors of sub-groups within a larger social group.

We can find other analogous examples of unusual language patterns in written forms by individuals we consider normative. However, we call those who produce them poets or authors. There are also innumerable instances of visual representations that are considered bizarre or non-comprehensible for some of us (e.g., Van Gogh, Cubist painters) but these individuals are considered artists, or sculptors, —not schizophrenics.

The same objections can be raised about the "appropriateness of affect" criteria. Does one require a different kind of explanation for the "expressive" or "effusive" response styles stereotypically attributed to women, in contrast to the "constrained" or "constricted" style stereotypically attributed to men? Would we look for genetic or bio-chemical substrate explanation? Is one or the other pathological? Would we think someone was "inappropriate" were she to say, while crying profusely at a wedding, "I'm so happy"; or "smiling" in a context more usually identified as a "frightening one"; or for someone (e.g., a male) being "stoic," unexpressive, or "controlled" in these same kinds of events?

Whenever a set of signs or symptoms has been identified for individuals diagnosed as schizophrenics, a large number of normal individuals have been found who also show the same sign or symptom pattern. To maintain the tradition, the claim is made that these nondiagnosed individuals have a sub-clinical, masked, latent, or atypical form of the pathology, or are "at risk," whatever these terms may denote or connote.

One counter-argument can be anticipated. The criteria for schizophrenia (or any of the other diagnostic categories) requires the concurrence of several of the disjunctive criteria, and these must persist for some time. Instances of signs or symptoms that persist for only a short time or that meet fewer that a criterial number of disjunctive criteria are not to be diagnosed. The grounds for requiring three symptoms, rather than two or four is unclear. Does meeting three criteria represent a distinct pathology, without regard to which three are met, or is it that individuals who show a greater difference in psychosocial transaction patterns are likely to be more disruptive for more people? Because the criteria are only partially correlated, it would not be unexpected to find large numbers of individuals who are not diagnosable, but act in ways consistent with one or the other of the designation criteria. One might even predict that there will be a greater number of individuals with one criterial action than there are with two and more with two than three. Here again the tradition is maintained by the claim that those with a lesser number of criterial actions are schizoid, latent, or incipient, or at risk for schizophrenia.

It is also unclear what is meant when someone is "at risk" for schizophrenia (or any other psychopathology). Does it mean anything other than that an observer can only identify less than the arbitrary number of disjunctive criteria used to diagnose? It is only if one believes that correlation means causation that one can even begin to use this kind of approach. That is, if there is a partial correlation of some action or attribute with those individuals who are diagnosed, then the assumption seems to be that each sign or symptom contributes to (causes) the "disease," or that the same underlying cause elicits each of the signs or symptoms, or that one is likely to get the disease if one does not watch out. Poverty is clearly a "risk" in this tradition.

Psychopharmacological and Neurological Arguments

The ostensible decrease in pathological behaviors after the administration of some psycho-pharmacological substance is often taken as evidence consistent with a medical-disease view. The argument here seems to be that if a psychopharmacological substance diminishes the atypical behaviors, no matter how different the kinds of psychosocial actions, it must be modifying some common underlying biological dysfunction. Although this argument is consistent with the concept of "syndrome" (an aggregation of a number of specific signs or symptoms which may or may not occur altogether in every instance), there is no evidence that all individuals who share the label "schizophrenic" (presumably sharing a syndrome) also respond favorably (or in the same way) to the ingestion of the same biochemical substance. Further, to the extent that individuals diagnosed quite differently (i.e., different syndromes and different diagnoses) do respond in a similar way to one pharmacological substance, and to the extent that all individuals with the same syndromes and diagnoses do *not* respond to the same biochemical substance, there seems to be some inconsistency, if not contradiction, in concluding that schizophrenia or any psychopathology (or their causes) can be identified reasonably by a common response to a biochemical substance. (See Wiener, 1989, for further discussion of this issue.)

Furthermore, if one chemical agent works for a while, and subsequently a different chemical agent is required in the treatment of the same individual, or if different biochemical agents show equivalent effects at different times, what shall we conclude about the pathologies in these different contexts? How is one to account for the waxing and waning of symptoms and for changes and variations in the behavior patterns of these defective, disrupted, deficient, disorganized individuals at different times and in different contexts, even though under all of these conditions they are taking the same medication (or taking no medication at all)?

Were one to find a one-to-one correspondence between biochemistry or neurology and a particular behavioral pattern, we would still face "the chicken or the egg" problem. Is the biochemistry or neurology the antecedent or the consequent, or only a correlate of particular psychosocial actions? Ekman (1983) has reported that individuals asked to behave *as if they were depressed* showed predictable and discriminable physiological pattern changes when they enacted the emotion. If such changes are correlated with *acting a behavior*, then one might question whether these kinds of physiological changes can be considered as evidence of a biological "cause" for the disease or syndrome.

Those who argue for a biological cause also seem to believe that the bio-physical-chemical substrate (e.g., brain and brain organization, gene, hormone) is prior to, and therefore the cause of, the "manifestation." One could well argue the contrary view, that much of brain organization is a function of the psychosocial activities of the person, and that early patterns of transactions with the socially organized world of objects, actions, contexts, and language (e.g., Clark & Holquist, 1984; Vygotsky, 1986), as well as the current ways a person acts in the world, can be said to account for the organization of the brain. That is, the kind and amount of activity (e.g., language and communication histories, learning, knowledge) are taken to contribute to current brain organization.

Although, there does appear to be some agreement that absence or removal of tissue limits the *range* of possible activities, there appear to be very few, if any, reliable reports of a one-to-one correspondence of any tissue locus with any complex psychosocial activity. As Salvador, Simon, Snay, and Llorens (1987) report, even with as basic a biological component as a hormone (i.e., testosterone in human males), there is a complex relationship between it and psycho-social actions (e.g., "competitive" fighting). They found that testosterone levels for their male "competitive" athlete subjects (in contrast to the non-competitive males in their sample) increased after exercise, but decreased slightly after competition. However, the more successful competitors showed an *increase* in their testosterone level after competition, whereas the less successful competitors showed a slight *decrease*. There was also a significant positive correlation between the degree of success in the past and the relative amount of inrease in the testosterone levels *after* the most recent competition.

Glosser, Wiener and Kaplan (1988) reported that individuals with identifiable left hemisphere tissue damage showed considerable inter-individual and remarkable *intra-individual* variability in communication patterns as a function of topic contents (e.g., "illness," family) and kind of communication modes (e.g., telephone, face-to-face, video system). There are also many anecdotal reports of brain damaged patients behaving quite differently in the hospital, at home, and in an experimental laboratory. It is difficult, if not impossible, to imagine a one-to-one correspondence of any biological event with any complex psychosocial action. The behavior - tissue relationship would seem to be more analogous to the *chicken and egg relationship*, i.e., a mutually interactive system, than to a simple causal model implied by the chemical intervention argument.

Genes

Cromwell (1984), in a systematic analysis of the relationship of genetic factors and schizophrenia, argued that any genetic heritability factor is likely to show only a very limited correlation, if any, with (1) one or the other of the very large number of behavioral forms now incorporated under the heterogeneous diagnostic category "schizophrenia" or (2) the psychosocial contexts in which the behaviors are viewed. Holtzman and Matthysse (1990) reviewed the many reports in the literature published since 1916 about the relationship of genetics and schizophrenia. They concluded that the "conventional approaches are not able to reveal anything about the ways genes influence that disorder, [and] that the family prevalence of schizophrenia is too low to fit a classical Mendelian transmission mode." They, like Cromwell, argue that a more fruitful approach would be to explore "genetic linkage" (e.g., some unusual perceptual events that seem to occur with many patients, labeled as "schizophrenic") rather than continuing to look for a direct genetic - schizophrenia relationship. However, Holtzman & Matthysse also cite Risch's comment that there is a "remarkable consistency of ... inconsistent findings in the recent history of linkage analyses of common psychiatric disorders" and Kendler's conclusion that "[unless we are] well informed of the difficulties and pitfalls ... linkage analysis could join the many scientific approaches to schizophrenia which have been characterized by rapid and overly enthusiastic endorsement by the psychiatric community—only to be followed by disappointment and precipitous rejection." Despite these caveats, and after rejecting current diagnostic classification as fruitless Holtzman and Matthysse continue to maintain the same genetic tradition when they argue that the study of the correlations of eye movement dysfunction for "schizophrenics and their probands" will make it possible to discover a genetic linkage. Since they also report that only 65% of schizophrenic patients (however these are identified) and only about 40% of their first degree relatives show the same "unusual" pattern of saccadic eye movements during tracking, the argument for genetic linkage does not seem very promising at this moment.

None of these arguments are about biological or other types of correlates of psychosocial actions. Rather, they are about questions of whether it is reasonable to believe that the kinds of biological events or other criteria that are being investigated can be considered to cause, explain, or identify what appear to be highly complex psychosocial actions. The issue here is that we continue to look for substrates for some kinds of atypical psychosocial transactions—those that are socially "disruptive"—but deem it unnecessary to use the same terms or arguments to explain the normative, typical, or usual psychosocial actions, or those atypical psychosocial actions that are socially facilitating.

Methodological Issues

There are also a number of methodological problems inherent in the empirical procedures used by investigators in this tradition to locate the population of concern to them. These investigators first select a schizophrenic population, using the disjunctive diagnostic criteria, each of which also incorporates considerable *heterogeneity* of psychosocial actions. This population of schizophrenics is then "matched" to some sample of normative (asymptomatic) individuals; a sample that is also quite heterogeneous. Four potential problems are quickly apparent in this paradigm. First, unless the identified behavior is evident for *all* individuals in the diagnosed schizophrenic sample, we are again faced with the problem of sub-groups. Second, if any of the normals show the ostensible commonality, we have still another problem. For example, what would be the consequences for clinical assessment if one were to find a behavior common to *all* of the schizophrenics, but also evident for a limited number of the normals (e.g., ten percent)? Using Meehl and Rosen's (1955) argument about the accuracy of prediction for low base-rate events, we get a very disconcerting outcome—regardless of whether the data come from diagnosis, risk factor, or genetic analyses. If schizophrenia occurs only once per hundred people in a population (as is claimed), then in a population of 1000, using these quite "discriminating" criteria (i.e., criteria that are met by 100% of "schizophrenics" and by only 10% of normative controls), we would identify the 10 schizophrenics *correctly*, but we would also identify 100 non-schizophrenics *incorrectly* as schizophrenics. Thus, even using such "ideal" empirical criteria, the results are that 10 times as many asymptomatic individuals are incorrectly identified; an outcome that makes it difficult to explain schizophrenia by exploring for a common underlying substrate. To maintain tradition, the claim is often made that these other individuals are at risk for schizophrenia, since all schizophrenics (at least in the experimental sample) show these criteria. (See Holzman & Matthysse, 1990, who make this claim explicitly.) In the convoluted logic of this claim the assertion "If Chinese, then the person drinks tea" becomes "If one drinks tea, then one is (or will become) Chinese." If we substitute schizophrenia as the antecedent, and the common behavior or the common substrate as the consequent, we can see the distortion in the risk-factor argument.

A second problem can be noted if one claims that what co-occurs with schizophrenia is its common substrate. If any relationship is found between schizophrenia and any other parameter, the most one can claim is a correlation (usually less than 1.0) of some aspects of the very complex behavioral patterns that are subsumed under schizophrenia, "patienthood" (e.g., isolation, hospitalization, medication), or the antecedents of "patienthood" (e.g., psychosocial history).

The third issue is a derivative of the second. What is an appropriate comparison group for schizophrenics? Ideally, this group should be equivalent in *all* aspects except for the criteria that designates one group as schizophrenic. Although it may be pragmatically difficult to match populations to this extent, one is always left with an unanswered question: are any of the differences that are found attributable to the schizophrenic/non-schizophrenic criteria, or are they a function of other factors that are partially correlated with "schizophrenic" (i.e., having been a patient, social class, education, language patterns, life styles, amount of social interaction, etc.).

We can recognize these kinds of problems most clearly if we explore the studies in which non-symptomatic patterns (e.g., eye tracking) of schizophrenic patients are contrasted with those of a normative control group. Some investigators in this tradition (e.g., Cromwell, 1984; Holtzman & Matthysse, 1990) argue that the primary requirement for now is to develop reliable criteria to identify homogeneous populations for clinicians and other investigators.

Although some of these investigators focus on "non-symptom" behavioral criteria (e.g., attention deficits, crossover reaction-time patterns) to help refine their "diagnostic" or selection criteria; they identify their target population by traditional psychiatric criteria, and seem to believe that once reliable populations are located, then it will be possible to find the common underlying (i.e., causal) substrate (i.e., genetic, or some other dysfunctional bio-physio-chemical system) by this procedure. Investigators using this approach are faced with exactly the same unresolved problems that confront the more obvious traditional approaches (with signs and symptoms).

Sociocultural Traditions

Although some investigators are concerned with sociocultural correlates or bases for labeling, more often than not they maintain the traditional metaphor of person dysfunction by claims that psychopathologies identify socioculturally defective, deficient, disrupted, or disorganized persons. Two subgroups can be identified in this sociocultural tradition. The focus for one group, for the most part, seems to be on an argument *against* the medical metaphor. These investigators claim that the behaviors in question are not necessarily physiochemically or biochemically linked, but are sociocultural labels for those individuals who are considered "difficult" for a social group. However, when these investigators continue to use such terms as "socially dysfunctional" (i.e., having problems in living in a particular society, being afflicted, or responding to anomie, or to forms of discrimination, etc.), they are explaining certain behaviors as if these were a different order of event than those we consider "adaptive." If one focuses on the deviant *person*, (i.e., one who performs certain atypical actions), then one sees that those who hold this perspective are not essentially different from the second group of investigators in the sociocultural tradition (e.g., Simons & Hughes, 1985), who argue that the sociocultural differences in schizophrenia are only *syndrome* differences, or only socially orchestrated variations of some (as yet unidentified) atypical, unusual, or universal substrate. It would seem that investigators in both of these subgroups—social construction approaches and syndrome difference approaches—remain committed to a different sort of explanation for typical actions than for psychosocial actions that are also culturally unusual. What seems to distinguish the social construction investigators from the traditional investigators is the different causes that they invoked to explain the "disruptive" behavioral occurrences.

An alternative view offered here is that "atypical" is to be understood as an arbitrary, normative-statistical notion; if the patterns of a population are explored, one will find a clear continuity within a group for any psychosocial action pattern. In the traditional approach, it is as if one is, in a sense, impelled to seek discontinuities for sociocultural categories. For example, in our culture we impose such subcategories as neonate, infant, toddler, pre-schooler, pre-teen, etc. (although other socio-cultural groups do not impose these distinctions), and then start to deal with individuals in these different categories as if there are clear and specifiable discontinuities among them (e.g., stages).

In the psychosocial approach, several different assumptions can be identified. The first is that *all* events that are considered behavioral are sociocultural manifestations, and every psychosocial action must of necessity include bodily correlates. An attempt to determine the primacy of these two concepts will lead to an indeterminate result; an analysis of psychosocial and biological events involves two different discourse systems. At best, one can only infer some order of correlation between the two sets of events. A second concern for investigators holding a psychosocial transaction view is the failure of traditional investigators to take into account the considerable *intra-individual* variability of psychosocial actions and biological events for all individuals in different contexts. With our current approaches to the study of psychosocial actions and of body action patterns, it is difficult to argue that either the psychosocial or biological discourse can explain the other. From a psychosocial transactional perspective, the focus is on the relationship of social interactions in an interpersonal social setting or context by individuals with particular psychosocial histories. Differences among individuals are explored in the same way we explore any differences that are deemed interesting by a sociocultural group (e.g., differences between men and women, the educated and the non-educated).

The basic arguments about such categories as schizophrenia, psychosis, and psychopathology are not about the facts or data or about one or another approach, (e.g., medical-disease, more reliable categorization, or social deviancy), but about the metaphor-paradigm that seems to permeate each of these approaches. These different perspectives seem to share a belief that whenever some set of psychosocial actions can be identified that is different from some arbitrary ideal; one can reasonably infer that there is something defective, deficient, disrupted, or disorganized about the person or of his or her action. Once a label is imposed, a different kind, sort, or class of explanation is offered for these kinds of atypical actions than is offered for the typical and the usual. Although the labels, criteria, conceptual framework, assumptions invoked for the unusual and atypical, and the kinds of instances specified as pathological, have changed over historical eras, even within the same sociocultural group; the current tradition has persisted.

What is an alternative to this traditional approach? As outlined in an analysis of depression (Wiener, 1989) and of anorexia (Marcus & Wiener, 1989), it may be helpful to explore first the diversity of instances that have been coordinated in the traditional framework. Then, if possible, one would explore these same instances as if one were a cultural anthropologist and did not "know" the native system. The attempt, then, is to determine what kinds of sociocultural commonalities or coordinates one can *impose* on the events, rather than on the person. At the same time, the "clinician-anthropologist" must always be alert to his or her highly acculturated biases that are brought to the observations and analyses. As anthropologists have noted repeatedly, "naive observation" is impossible when one recognizes that every observer is a member of a particular sociocultural group with a particular psychosocial history. The best one can do, given the proposed framework, is to *construct* a biography (case study) in psychosocial action terms within the confines of an *explicit* conceptual metaphor and paradigm (disciplinary matrix), without assuming a realist philosophical perspective, a perspective that seems pervasive in almost all traditional approaches.

References

American Psychiatric Association (1987). *Diagnostic and statistical manual of mental disorders,* 3rd ed., revised. Washington, DC.

Baker, E. (1986). *Categorization of natural objects by aphasics and non-brain-damaged adults: An experimental analysis of featured dimensions.* Unpublished doctoral dissertation, Clark University, Worcester, MA.

Black, (1954). Metaphor. *Aristotelian Society Proceedings, 55,* 284-285.

Cantor, N., Smith, E.E., French-deSales, R., & Mezzich, J. (1980). Psychiatric diagnosis as prototype categorization. *Journal of Abnormal Psychology, 89,* 181-193.

Clark, K., & Holquist, M. (1984). *Mikhail Bakhtin.* Cambridge, MA: Harvard University Press.

Cloninger, R.C., Martin, R.L., Guze, S.B., & Clayton, P.J. (1985). Diagnosis and prognosis in schizophrenia. *Archives of General Psychiatry, 42,* 15-25.

Cromwell, R. (1984). Preemptive thinking and schizophrenic research. In W.I. Spaulding & J.E. Cole (Eds.), *Theories of schizophrenia & psychosis.* Nebraska symposium on motivation. Lincoln, NE: University of Nebraska Press.

Ekman, P. (1983). Autonomic nervous system activity distinguishes among emotion. *Science, 221,* 1208-1210.

Glosser, G., Wiener, M., & Kaplan, E. (1988). Variations in aphasic language behaviors. *Journal of Speech and Hearing Disorders, 53,* 115-124.

Goodwin, D.W., & Guze, S.B. (1984). *Psychiatric diagnosis* (3rd ed.). New York: Oxford University Press.

Guze, S.B. (1970). The need for toughmindedness in psychiatric thinking. *Southern Medical Journal, 63,* 661-671.

Holzman, P.S. & Matthysse, S. (1990). The genetics of schizophrenia: A review. *Psychological Science, 1,* 279-286.

Kendell, R.E. (1975). *The role of diagnosis in psychiatry.* Oxford: Blackwell Scientific Publications.

Kendell, R.E. (1982). The choice of diagnostic criteria for biological research. *Archives of General Psychiatry, 39,* 1334-1339.

Kendell, R.E. (1986). The concept of disease and its implications for psychiatry. In A. Kerr & P. Snaith (Eds.), *Contemporary issues in schizophrenia.* Avon: The Bath Press.

Kerr, A. & Snaith, P. (Eds.). (1986). *Contemporary issues in schizophrenia.* Avon: The Bath Press.

Kuhn, T.S. (1972). *The structure of scientific revolutions* (2nd ed.). Chicago: The University of Chicago Press.

Landrine, H. (1989). The social class-schizophrenia relationship: A different approach and new hypothesis. *Journal of Social and Clinical Psychology, 8,* 288-303.

Marcus, D. & Wiener, M. (1989). Anorexia nervosa reconceptualized from a Psychosocial Transactional perspective. *American Journal of Orthopsychiatry, 59*(3), 346-384.

Meehl, P. & Rosen, A. (1955). Antecedent probability and the efficiency of psychometric signs, patterns, or cutting scores. *Psychological Bulletin, 52,* 194-216.

Rosch, E.N. (1978). Principles of categorization. In E.N. Rosch & B.B. Lloyd (Eds.), *Cognition and categorization.* Hillsdale, NJ: Erlbaum.

Ryle, G. (1949). *The concept of mind.* New York: Barnes & Noble Books.

Salvador, A., Simon, V., Snay, F., & Llorens, L. (1987). Testosterone and cortisol responses to competitive fighting in human males: A pilot study. *Aggressive Behavior, 13,* 9-13.

Sarbin, T.R. (1967). The concept of hallucination. *Journal of Personality, 35,* 359-380.

Scheff, T.J. (1966). *Being mentally ill: A sociological theory.* Chicago: Aldine.

Scheff, T.J. (1974). The labeling theory of mental illness. *American Sociological Review, 39,* 444-452.

Simon, R.C. & Hughes, C.C. (Eds.). (1985). *The culture-bound syndrome.* Boston: Reidel.

Smith, E.E., Balzant, G.J., & Walker, J. (1978). Nominal, perceptual and semantic codes in picture categorization. In J.W. Cotton & R.L. Klatsky (Eds.), *Semantic factors in cognition.* Hillsdale, NJ: Erlbaum.

Smith, E.E. & Medin, D.L. (1981). *Categories and concepts.* Cambridge: Harvard University Press.

Smith, E.E., Shoben, E.J., & Rips, L.J. (1974). Structure and process in semantic memory: A featured model for semantic discrimination. *Psychological Review, 81,* 214-241.

Spaulding, W.D., & Cole, J.K. (Eds.). (1984). *Theories of schizophrenia & psychosis.* Nebraska symposium on motivation. Lincoln, NE: University of Nebraska Press.

Tajfel, H. (Ed.). (1978). *Differentiation between social groups.* London: Academic Press.

Tajfel, H., Sheikh, A.A., & Gardner, R.C. (1964). Content of stereotypes and the inference of similarity between members of stereotyped groups. *Acta Psychologia, 22,* 191-201.

Tajfel, H. & Wilkes, A.L. (1963). Classification and quantitative judgement. *British Journal of Psychology, 54,* 101-114.

Turbayne, C.M. (1970). *The myth of the metaphor* (revised edition). Columbia, SC:

University of South Carolina Press.

Vygotsky, L. (1986). *Thought and Language* (A. Kozulin, Translator). Cambridge, MA: The MIT Press.

Wiener, M. (1989). Psychopathology reconsidered: Depression interpreted as psychosocial transactions. *Clinical Psychology Review, 9,* 295-321.

Woodruff, R.A., Goodwin, D.W., & Guze, S.B. (1974). *Psychiatric diagnosis* (1st ed.). New York: Oxford University Press.

15
A War of Words? A War of Worlds? The Struggle over the Definition of Schizophrenia

Bernard Kaplan

On the program listing the performances that were to constitute a large part of this "international conference," of which this volume is the outcome, I found myself charged with presenting a paper entitled *Current critiques of the concept of schizophrenia.* I could not recall whether I had casually tossed out that title myself (I had) or whether it had been foisted on me by the organizers of the conference, caught between my typical resistance to titling a paper before I had finished it and publicity-generated demands for a list of titles for a program far in advance of the actual occasion. In any case, that original title did not quite represent either what I intended to, or finally did, speak about.

Doubtless, some will be able to find in my chapter the greatly refracted influence of several of those who have, in recent years, raised or resurrected questions about cultural and discursive practices into which the terms *schizophrenia* and *schizophrenic*, as well as the putative referents of such terms, have found their way. I refer here, among others, to Szasz (1970; 1974) and Sarbin and Mancuso (1980), among others, who had trained their torpedos directly at the term and concepts of schizophrenia. But those who have far more strongly influenced my thinking on these matters (e.g., neo-Marxists, radical feminists, culture critics) have never written directly about *schizophrenia* or *schizophrenics* (although some had discussed madness), but have rather raised general questions about constructions of reality; about "authority" and "legitimation" in the representation of what there is; about the politics of representation and interpretation; about power and its relation to "knowledge;" about "structures of dominance," which allow voice and the dissemination of opinions on contestable issues to certain groups and enforce the muteness of others.

In sum, I have not here taken it upon myself to represent and mediate the views of others, who can speak eloquently for themselves. Rather, informed by the insights of these and other others, I hope to highlight a number of issues and raise a series of questions provoked by the framing of the conference itself, the election of participants for the conference, the projected format of the conference, and the topics foregrounded by the organizers of the conference. I will begin by focussing on the structure and supposed function of the conference itself. I will then use the original prospectus for the conference as a kind of "agent provocateur" to raise more "substantive" questions.

Doubtless affected by my own latent paranoia, or by a character disease which some expert might designate as *folie de doute*, I am inclined to suppress my tendencies toward instant credulity, especially where someone in power or authority undertakes or proposes some action "in the national interest" or for attaining some universally beneficial goal. This is not to suggest that I will actively resist going along with the mob in some circumstances, but only to acknowledge that I am afflicted by other, counter voices as I do so.

I mention this here because—despite my acceptance of the invitation to participate in the conference—I had wondered, sotto voce and even publically, why a conference on schizophrenia, (especially one with the overarching title, "What is schizophrenia?") had been convened at this time. Were there any momentous events on the national or international scene (e.g., like the spread of AIDS or the collapse of the Soviet system) which might warrant a "conference?" Were there any in-house novelties of vision calling for a radical reexamination of the entire 'field' of thinking and research in "schizophrenia?"

More than thirty years ago, Silvano Arieti, generally recognized as a major figure in the "field of schizophrenia," in one of his articles on *schizophrenia* in his *American Handbook of Psychiatry*, summarized the outcome of sessions at the Second International Congress for Psychiatry, devoted entirely to "this disorder":

> There was not a single concept on schizophrenia [advanced by any of the attendant psychiatrists] that was not rejected or challenged by some other authors. Even the name schizophrenia was disapproved by several people. (1959, p. 455, my insert)

Since that time, there have surely been many conferences devoted entirely to that "disorder," and many books published representing the diverse and conflicting points of view expressed at that international congress. There have even been books raising questions about the conception of schizophrenia as a "disease'; especially as a disease or disorder amenable to 'diagnosis' and 'treatment' by that special professional guild called psychiatrists, or any other "mental health" experts. Is there any indication that these questions and critiques have been confronted by professionals "in the field" other than an occasional acknowledgment that they have been voiced, followed by a quick return to business as usual? It is noteworthy that Arieti, whom even Thomas Szasz (1976), in his near universal excoriation of psychiatrists, credits with a "fundamental decency," goes on, blithely, to promote the ontologization of schizophrenia and a schizophrenic syndrome, even while conceding that what is said about this putative process is "indefinite, variable, inconstant." He opines (feels):

> that there is a more or less homogeneous core which makes *us* recognize the schizophrenic person as such and leads *us* to *some conclusions, some of which have pragmatic value.* The fact that the nature of this core has not yet been fully or uncontroversially determined points to the incompleteness of the concept of schizophrenia, but does not prove it a fallacy. (1959, p. 501, italics mine)

It is not my central point here that the same kind of "intuitive" certainty has been invoked to establish the widespread "objective" existence of demons and witches in earlier times, communist sympathizers during the McCarthy era, and enemies of the state on all occasions; or that "conclusions" which one is led to by such objectified entities have always had *some* 'pragmatic value,' e.g., the recognition, by the discerning eyes of the experts in such matters, of some *homogeneous core*, taken as *inherent* or *intrinsic* to the entities thus recognized, has invariably led, in different cultural contexts, to diverse proposals for practical action, such as burning, incarcerating, torturing, and defaming.

My central point here/now is rather the following: if Arieti, whom I knew personally to be not only a remarkably decent individual—but also widely read, erudite, cultured, and open to new ideas—was able to resist, or so easily discount, the kinds of criticisms launched by Szasz and others, why would one believe that there would be less resistance today to any fundamental questioning of the long-standing reification and objectification of *schizophrenia* and *schizophrenics* among the typical members of the psychiatric and clinical-psychological guilds who, after all, have much of their *raison d'etre* in their presumed special capacity to diagnose and treat "mental diseases?" I intend nothing invidious in this question. All of us, trained in certain practices and ways of thinking and talking, and rewarded as well as protected by our institutionalized "disciplines" and professions; are likely to suffer, as Burke (1935), following Dewey, would say, from our *occupational psychoses;* representing, describing, interpreting what confronts us in terms of our sedimented prejudices.

Given the likelihood that, once again, well-entrenched "prejudices" of each of us would be rehearsed, I puzzled over what could be the intended function of this kind of conference at this time. It was surely not intended as one of those conferences designed for the exchange of *information.* Nor did it appear likely to be one of those meetings, like a House-Senate Conference, in which differences would be negotiated and mutual compromises made, to arrive at some position grudgingly acceptable to all sides. The controversial issues here were too deeply felt, like the issues separating advocates of *right-to-life* from advocates of *free choice.*

One can scarcely expect that those who, "before reading" (see Rabinowitz, 1989) take it for granted that *schizophrenia* designates some naturally occurring happening—an event whose cause or causes (biological, psychological, "psychodynamic," sociological) will eventually be discovered in the realm of pristine Nature—will find some point of negotiation and compromise with those who might suggest, with Foucault (1961), and perhaps Sarbin and Mancuso (1980), that it is one terminological component of a set of discursive practices, used by groups in power to subjugate, subordinate, "pathologize-medicalize," and, if possible or convenient, *normalize.* Nor would we expectthem to agree with those who deviate from the values and norms of a social order; who would insist, with Szasz (1970; 1976), and perhaps Sarbin/Mancuso, that *schizophrenia* is a politico-axiological epithet, invented and perpetuated by psychiatrists and their cortége under the mystifying pretense of denoting some natural, objective process, amenable to 'scientific' description and explanation; or who would hunker down, with Wiener, (this volume) and insist that *schizophrenia* is a term *sans* meaning or reference.

The schism here is far too deep. It goes far beyond the issue of different "philosophies of science." It involves basic divergences in Weltanschauungen or orientations, in which the very nature and status of what we take to be *reality, knowledge,* and *science* are always already in dispute.

Assuming and anticipating, as I had, such a state of affairs, I had hoped that something of significance might be salvaged through the format of the conference. Perhaps the conference organizers would arrange for rip-roaring debates between the advocates of antipodal positions, through which a potential reader of the proceedings of this convocation (ostensibly in limbo as to how to think about "schizophrenia") could be exposed to the rough and tumble of full-scale dialogues. Or, perhaps there would be round-table discussions, without prepared papers, in which theses advanced by any one participant would be open to challenge and dispute by others. But, even if such explosive formats were implicitly considered by the conference organizers, they did not occupy the center ring of the circus.

Instead, we were, in general, blessed with one more instance of the now "traditional" format for academic and professional conferences and symposia, in which different speakers briefly present their diverse points of view to a more or less tolerant audience, entertain a few questions and comments, with a final "discussant" called upon to summarize, "synthesize" and/or criticize what he/she has taken the prior speakers in the "session" to have said. One was reminded of one of those television shows, like Nightline, in which one listens first to Shamir and then to Arafat, or first to a passionate advocate of "right-to-life" and then, to an equally passionate advocate for "free choice," with the moderator serving as interlocutor. Such an arrangement was scarcely calculated to foster the kinds of arguments and deep explorations with respect to deeply felt issues which occur in the world outside of the academy. To be sure, there were occasional flare-ups, despite the format; but, in general, the kind of enervating 'civility' and concern for proper order, which mark typical symposia precluded a knock-down, drag-out debate, or any deep discussion of the radically different presuppositions governing the discourse.

Although much more may be said about the framing of this conference, I shall conclude my prologue with a note about the selection of participants. I surely appreciate the fact that anyone organizing a conference may have considerable difficulty in securing a representative of *all* of the groups who might be taken to have some involvement and interest in the topic. One may have tried to recruit such representatives and been turned down for any number of reasons. Nevertheless, irrespective of the validity of the reasons, it stands out like the proverbial sore thumb that there were no women or, better, feminists among the participants; no cultural or intellectual historians; and no representatives of the 'group' whose presumed 'illness' or 'disease' was the ostensible object of discussion (See Knapp, 1986). Nor was there any representative of the Jungian group of 'therapists' (e.g., J.W. Perry), whose conceptions of the nature of mind (psyche) and reality are decidedly at variance with all of those present.

Surely, we have become aware, or should have become aware, over the past three decades, of the fact that many of those who have been rubricized under socio-cultural headings, in terms of objectified properties pertaining to race, gender, sexual preference, political status, etc., have turned against their surveyors and self-designated benign protectors. They have often recognized that their 'circumdescription' by others, their dislocation to a denigrated/stigmatized category, was not in their interest, but rather served the interests of those who had thus categorized them. We have seen the bitter attacks of formerly (or still) marginalized or muted groups not only against the powerful forces which have malevolently marginalized them, but also against we establishment "liberals," who claimed to speak on their behalf or to work disinterestedly, in their interests. (See Bayer, 1987)

I will not speculate here about the reasons or motives governing the formation of the invited guest list for this party, on the rationales or rationalizations for inclusion and exclusion. I simply wish to emphasize that this is an issue that calls for close examination whenever a conference is called on some "momentous" topic, especially when the conveners of the conference emphasize their desire to insure diversity and an equal voice for all or even only for all concerned *professionals*.

I have spent so much time on preliminaries because I have learned from T.S. Eliot and Edward Said that in one's beginning is one's end. The way in which a conference is framed, the selection of participants, the formatting of the program, the very titling of the topic, *incline* us in a certain direction, even if they do not *necessitate* that we follow that direction.

I turn now to the prospectus for the conference *proper* and to the questions issued by the organizers of this convocation to direct our attention and intention.

It will not have escaped notice that the very title of the conference is ambiguous. Were we asked to assume that *schizophrenia* is some actual process, event, or happening in the world, and requested to give our various characterizations of this putative existent, our different ways of representing *what it is*, like the blind men with the elephant in the well-known fable? Or were we asked to give our several definitions of the *term*, *schizophrenia*, irrespective of any issue of reference to some independent existent, much as we might manifest our lexicographic skills in answering the questions, "What is a centaur?, What is a demon?, What is phlogiston?" I don't want to get here into the sharp and cogent criticisms raised by Quine and others about the warrant for any radical diremption between analytic and synthetic statements. It suffices to say that, in most contexts, we can distinguish between a request for a description of some object and a request for a definition of some expression.

Few here, I would suppose, believe that those who use the terms, *schizophrenia* or *schizophrenic* have nothing in mind in using those terms or simply use them as a panchreston or an epithet of disapproval; although some may question whether those who use the terms are consistent or unequivocal in their usage; they may also question whether there is anything in our *actual* world (as opposed to possible or fictional worlds) denoted by those terms.

It would seem from the prospectus that one or more of the organizers presupposed that there were "objective" phenomena designated by the terms, just as Arieti had earlier presupposed that there were "objective" processes and entities corresponding to the terms, even though what was predicated of those existent phenomena by diverse investigators was "indefinite, variable and inconstant." Thus we are early informed, with some tone of dismay, that:

> Many investigators of schizophrenia agree that a major stumbling block to progress [sic] in the field [sic] is the lack of a single definition of the *phenomenon* which is acceptable to everyone concerned.

One may note in passing that this statement presupposes that there is not only a word, but also a self-subsistent phenomenon to be defined. Why, it may be asked, should one assume, to borrow Quine's quaint formula, that "ontology recapitulates philology;" that the presence of a name in discourse entails the "objective" existence of something denoted by the name? One would scarcely say today, with regard to angelology or demonology, that a major block to progress in these fields is the lack of a single definition of the *phenomenon*, which is acceptable to everyone concerned.

Indeed, with regard to some equally unspecified notion of "progress in a field," it might be said that a full realization of the diverse meanings given to terms or conceptions like *angel* and *demon* in different cultural, political, and economic contexts may constitute a greater contribution to progress than any coercive attempt to cabin, crib, and confine the meaning of those terms. To be sure, this practice would bracket or suspend the search for a transcendent signified or referent, and focus on the use of such terms as *symbolic actions* (Burke) employed in various ways by different agents operating in different scenes for different ends or purposes. A project of this kind, with regard to *madness*, has been pursued by Foucault (1961).

Now, since issues of "definition" recur throughout the prospectus, it may be of some value to ask ourselves what is involved in definition in general and in the definition of schizophrenia in particular. One should not, of course, assume here that definition has a single function. We may note from the Oxford English Dictionary (OED) that *define* is glossed as "to determine the boundary or spatial extent of; to settle the limits of," and is used figuratively as well as "literally." In another acceptation, *define* is paraphrased as "to determine, lay down definitely, fix; decide; decide upon." Related to this specification, we have *define* as "determining, deciding upon." The word is also glossed as "to state precisely or determinately; to specify; to state exactly what a thing is; to set forth the essential nature of; to state the nature and properties of."

If we turn to *definition*, we note here again an emphasis on (someone) setting boundaries or limits. Of special interest perhaps is the conception of definition: "the action of determining a controversy or question at issue; specifically a formal decision or pronouncement of an *ecclesiastical authority*." (my emphasis).

Now, it should be apparent from these various glosses on *defining* and *definition* that defining is often, if not always, one component of an agonistic *act*; it is part and parcel of a scene of conflict between opposing agents, even where, in many cases, there is an asymmetry of power between the protagonists. One may see this clearly, on a "literal" level, where it is an issue of demarcating one area of land from another, of defining one's territory or property. One may not see this quite so clearly when the issue is one of demarcating one "thing" from another or one class of things from others. One may be even less aware of it (on the so-called "figurative" level) in cases in which there is a conflict over the 'meanings' to be assigned to terms. Nevertheless, as Burke has noted, in *all* defining, there is an element of *fiat*: Let that be X! Let that be called X! (For a profound treatment of issues of definition, see Burke, 1945, Chapter 2.)

We can all, perhaps, understand a passion for setting bounds and limits; such a process enables us to mark off one thing from another or one class of things from another, the grouping ostensibly dependent on our interests and purposes. If we have different interests and purposes, we will mark off, or attempt to mark off, the world differently. From this perspective, it is absurd to ask for a definition—a definitive definition—of anything including reality or schizophrenia one which will end all discussion of differences in this matter, all attempts to overthrow the regnant definition. Actual and potential revisionists, like termites, are always in the woodwork. Of course, one can always bring in an 'ecclesiastical authority' or some analogous secular body to utter definitive pronouncements as to the way things are and the fixed meanings that terms are to have. Those who diverge from the authoritative pronouncement will then be imprisoned, exiled, or obliged to take hemlock.

Once one foregrounds the *fiat* character of *all* definitions and the inescapable contestation between different groups over what W.I. Thomas, many years ago, called "the definition of the situation", (a contestation manifested here in the struggle over the definition of "schizophrenia") one may be prompted to ask the Burkean questions: *Who* defines? in what *scene*? with what *Instrumentalities* ("definitions" may be insinuated into discourse and practice in various ways)? for what *goals* or *purposes*? One may ask, further, "Whose definitions of situations, "things," "processes," etc., become dominant or gain hegemony in a social order of multiple voices?" "How do certain groups gain the power and authority to foist their definitions of situations on others?" "What attitudes and actions are evoked by such definitions?" "In whose interests are such definitions?" "Which groups profit from such definitions?" "Which groups suffer from them?" Such questions, and many others like them, take us away from the issue of "veridical" or faithful representation of what there is independent of all "knowers," and lead us to focus on the *politics* and *rhetoric* involved in the joint and conflictful constitution of our Lebenswelt.

One of the reasons I called attention earlier to the absence of any feminist among the participants in this conference is that, in recent decades it has been feminists who have persistently and recurrently called attention to the political character of *naming, defining*, and *classifying* the world and its "constituents." Speaking not only for themselves, but for other muted groups who have been denigrated, defamed, oppressed, (radical) feminists have insisted that we not only examine our sedimented representations of *what there is*, but also recognize their provenance and struggle to change them.(See Lloyd, 1989; Riley, 1989)

Relatedly, one of the reasons why I earlier remarked on the absence of an intellectual (or social) historian in this conference is my conviction that most, if not all, of our current terms and conceptions have their roots in history, even though their historical provenance may have been occulted or ignored. Where such obscuration occurs, we are typically inclined to reify and essentialize or eternalize the putative referents of such terms and concepts, and endow them with an 'autonomy' or self-subsistence; forgetting that the term or concept was introduced, perpetuated, and disseminated by certain groups with certain orientations and interests, and for certain purposes. A good intellectual (or social) historian would oblige us to remember.

In this connection, it may be interesting, especially when there is so much emphasis by some of the conference conveners on *theory*, and the need for adequate *theory* with regard to schizophrenia, if we are to make progress 'in the field,' to note the provenance of the term, "theory,". If one indulges an amateur penchant for etymology, one finds that our exalted term derives from the institution of the *theoros* in ancient Greece, a specially selected group (analogous to our experts and professionals, or to what Znaniecki once referred to as "men of knowledge") whose role it was to provide *the* authoritative definition/representation of certain situations for subsequent *public* discourse, thereby marginalizing or obliterating other voices (those of *hoi polloi*) whose representations of what had happened could then be taken to be idiosyncratic and hence dismissible, except as an occasion for local gossip. Is it surprising that different theorists still seek, and are often permitted, to preempt or usurp the categories of public discourse; to stipulate how events and situations are to be defined, described, or represented, to be articulated and 'explained?'

If I may hazard an "armchair, partisan, diagnosis," it seems to me that those investigators who are preoccupied with the lack of a single canonical definition and monolithic overarching theory of schizophrenia, and who take such diversity and seeming cacophony to be "a stumbling block" to some kind of unspecified progress in some nominally demarcated but otherwise unspecified field, are mainly disturbed (dis-eased, dis-organized, confused) by an unwillingness of, or resistance by, others to adopt *their* definition or theory of the putative phenomenon. An "arm-chair, Kraeplinian, prognosis" as to the inevitable course of this disease: after having 'demonstrated' to their own satisfaction the errors and limitations of all other claimants to define and theorize the "field," they will proudly announce their own formulae for restoring law and order.

It seems to have been the preoccupation of one or more of the conference organizers that unless all of us or, at least, all of us *professionals*, are able to arrive at a single, unequivocal, universally acceptable, *definition* of the "snark" (schizophrenia), we shall continue to flounder around—speaking at cross-purposes, each using 'definitions' consistent with his/her particular theoretical "bias"—or be obliged to "opt for a purely empirical approach as encompassed in the DSM-III-R." In this preoccupation there lurks a postivist presupposition that there can be such a phenomenon as a non-theoretical or purely empirical definition, a definition from no point of view or a God's eye point of view, that directly represents things "as they are, and not upon a blue guitar." I will refrain from commenting on the invocation of the "ecclesiastic authority", DSM-III-R, as the ultimate arbiter of such a "purely empirical definition."

Now, doubtless, if we are to escape an attenuated version of the phenomenon of "beireden," which is sometimes taken as a "diagnostic sign" or "symptom" of *schizophrenia,* we (whoever *we* are in a dialogue, conversation or controversy) will feel the need for some consensus about a foundation, a stable 'definition' on which we can, in specific contexts, agree, before we take off from that common basis either further to agree, or to agree to disagree. It is, I believe, this need for a common starting point that leads to demands for "purely empirical" or "operational" definitions and/or for a description of the *whats* at issue, severed from "explanatory or causal accounts" which attempt to provide *whys* for the *whats*.

This communication requirement for a common denominator should not be taken to imply that the *whats* are unproblematic or available to the intuitions of Everyman, irrespective of history or acculturation; that they themselves are "theory-free." Every *what*, ostensibly denoted by ostension ("there's one, there's another!"), must still enter discourse via some *representation*, and the representations of seemingly given *whats* may differ for different societies, different groups, and different individuals. Thus, the presumed *what* which Kraepelin designated/ described as *dementia praecox* was not the same *what* that Bleuler designated/described as *schizophrenia*. Nor, as we are well aware, is the putative *what*, designated/denoted as *schizophrenia*, the same *what* for each of the designators/denoters.

Given this state of affairs, it is an act of presumption, credulity, or cooptation by the 'metaphysics of presence,' to assert, as some have, that there is, in ontology, something *out* there with a "common core," that can be unequivocally identified in every society and in every historical period.

This presumption that it is possible to denote or designate an individual entity or class of entities, prior to, and independent of, their representation in discourse (that's an X, there's another X) and that politics, rhetoric and language enter after an intuition of essences, has often (alas all too often) led to the procedure of corralling a group of entities together as presumed members of a "natural kind," and then seeking "inductively" or "experimentally" to arrive at the discriminating features which will suffice to mark off (define) that group from any other group.

As we surely have seen with the Everest of 'research' on *schizophrenia*, (See Bellak, 1979) such a gathering of physically contoured beings into a single class on the basis of their presumed *essential similarity* leads to the surprising (to some) realization that the *evidence* (a term/concept also taken as unproblematic and theory-neutral) *shows* that the segregated group whose common essence had been intuited, has no distinctive properties or set of properties that warrant the segregation of that group from other groups.

Such a depressing "finding" which is unlikely to stymie those who are convinced that there is a Holy Grail *out there*, may prompt the weak of faith to reconsider their presuppositions and The Way (met-hodos) they have chosen. Some may come to the conclusion that they must decide, *beforehand*, what they intend by the term/concept *schizophrenia* (as well as the entire field of terms with which they wish to contrast *schizophrenia*), and only then seek to ascertain whether there are any "phenomena" in their actual world that can be taken by them and others to exemplify what they mean. In this way, they would subscribe to the Copernican revolution initiated by Kant and further articulated by the neo-Kantians (Cohen, Rickert, Cassirer, et al.).

In such a *con*version (which some may take as a *per*version due to the hegemony of mathematics in "natural science" inquiry), one moves from traditional substance concepts to function concepts; from atomic items in simple location to a field in which the status, value, and significance of an element depends upon the field or structure of which it is a part, and with which it is indissociably connected. (See Bergner, 1988; Cassirer, 1944; 1953). Of course, this displacement from intuited substances to the system of epistemic categories introduced, "through the free play of the imagination" by the "scientific" investigator may easily wreak havoc with our everyday denotations and classifications, our *social* construction of reality (See Berger & Luckmann, 1967). What God hath there seemingly united is now divorced; and intuitively given segregated items are now seen as variants of a one, or as epiphenomena of an underlying "true" reality (See Baker, 1987).

On the other hand, the tension between what F.S.C. Northrop has called *concepts by intuition* (everyday descriptors, such as insect, fish, table, crazy, etc.) and *concepts by postulation* (scientific terms, such as mass, force, electron, quark, etc.) may lead others, who may have been initially seized by the fancy of an Icarian voyage, to experience an access and excess of vertigo; they may decide to forego leaving the cave, and seek to hug the Earth (Lebenswelt, the everyday given reality). But now with the realization that the objects of this everyday actuality are not natural *givens*, immaculately perceived by any innocent eye. They are, rather, *anthropocentric, politico-culturally constructed, parochial* entities; part of one *socially constituted ontology*, which may differ radically from other socially constructed ontologies.

Whether it is possible for human beings at any time or place to arrive at the way things are in themselves, independent of the myths grounding the socio-cosmic "order" into which each of us is thrust; free of the fears, wishes, desires, and values which afflict all of us; is not an issue I will discuss here. In this unknown realm, which is sometimes baptized as the Really Real or the Out There, presumptively all would be in flux, or everything would be what it is, and not some other thing (or event); such distinctions which we find useful, even inescapable, in our everyday worlds such as *healthy* or *diseased, ordered* or *disordered, integrated* or *disintegrated, sane* or *insane, weeds, trash,* or *heresies,* etc., would not obtain. Nor would there be any of the other Nama and Rupa (names and forms)—the offspring of *Maya*—instituted by human beings in their attempts to cope with existence. Like poems in Archibald MacLeish's *Ars Poetica*, events would not *mean*, but only *be*.

This is not the case in our *socially constituted* ontology, nor do we know of any society in which it is or has been the case. Everywhere, in terms of human interest—we may provisionally adopt Habermas' generic types of interest—processes are reified or hypostatized, classifications (taxonomies, nosologies) are instituted, definitions are imposed to segregate certain phenomena from others, and various relations are asserted between classes of entities distinguished from other classes. Norms and standards are introduced to establish the diverse *whats* of the world, and to help us in re-marking both deviations from the paradigm cases of each of the *what's,* or the dangerous liminal areas (that which is neither fish nor fowl, male nor female) between demarcated *whats* (See Douglas, 1966; 1982; Turner, 1967, 1974).

All of this, of course, has been observed mainly by sophisticated, secular, professional anthropologists and others as *spectators, outside* the sociocultural orders which they research and investigate: by "scientists" who take God or the gods to have died or never to have been. Such scholars have also informed us that, *within* so called primitive or primary oral societies, and even in presumptively more "advanced" societies, the *Order of Nature*, including the various distinctions among categories of things and events, and the various prescriptions and proscriptions as to what one should expect from, and how one should act toward, the various kinds of distinguished things and events, are taken to have been established, once and for all, by founding deities *in illo tempore* (Eliade), and not by human beings working with and against other human beings to live, live well and live better. A somewhat attenuated version of this kind of cosmogonic vision is that in which a personified Nature or a depersonalized evolutionary process establishes diverse *natural kinds* (species)—kinds in which the members share certain *essential* properties in common, whatever the *accidental* variations they may manifest, which serve to individuate them.

Now, I am one of those secularized human beings, who believes that the structures, orders, or organizations of our worlds are not given to us from on high (or *ab extra*) by some deities who knew how to carve at the joints, but have been constituted, dissolved, reconstituted, and altered by human beings, in episodic cooperation and conflict with other human beings, throughout history, through their various actions and their diverse discursive practices.

From this point of view, the ways in which phenomena are *represented*; acts of *identifying* things, events, processes, persons; *classifying* sets of things, events, etc.; *dividing* things, events, persons from other things, events, persons; *relating* entities to each other in various ways; *hierarchizing* or *stratifying* the various classes which are distinguished, etc., are not the dispassionate activities of contemplative seers, penetrating and descrying the God-given order of Nature, a mimesis of what there is. They are, rather, passionate *proposals* to construe the world in certain ways instead of others, not for oneself or one's group alone, but for everyone.

Through a "social amnesia" or diverse processes of mystification, the human and conflictful origin of such proposals is occulted, and certain orders or patterns of organization are taken to be natural, normal—essentially the way things are. Any deviation in action or expression from such a putatively natural order is taken as a harbinger of Chaos or Anarchy, in which "things fall apart" *because* the "centre does not hold." As we "know," the agents invoked to account for recurrent Decline and Falls of the House of Essence (the presumed natural order of things) have included Satan, the Devil, internal enemies, external enemies, etc. It is in this context, I believe, that the representation of some phenomena as "diseases" enters the picture. As I noted before, there are no diseases in that hypothetical ontology transcending all social ontologies, all social constructions of reality.

It is only from an anthropocentric and/or sociocentric viewpoint, in which certain norms are posited or taken for granted, that one may characterize, not only what is called cancer, multiple sclerosis, pneumonia, syphilis, etc. as diseases (or disorders), but also what is called "schizophrenia." One might even refer, in certain social groups, to hurricanes, tornados or earthquakes as "diseases" or "disorders" (for us, of course, such an extended usage could only be "figurative") insofar as they are taken to violate desiderata as to the way the cosmos ought to operate.

What is a "disease," or better, what do we take to be a disease? As is my wont, I went to the OED to check on the presumed etymology of the term. The emphasis there was on "discomfort," but it was soon used to refer to any phenomenon that is construed as a deviation from order or from an optimal state of health. Although not in this canonical source of lexical genealogies, I did, in another etymological handbook, come across a different origin of *disease*, one that suggested that it was born in the House of Essences. Before being claimed by the Aesclepiads and their descendants, *disease* was used, according to this source, to pertain to *any* deviation from the presumed essence or the 'natural kind' to which a thing or event was taken to belong: *dis-esse*—a privation of the (true) being or nature of that entity.

Whether or not that lineage can be legitimatized or merely relegated to the category of bastardy, it is obvious that the term *disease* has been widely used to designate negatively valorized deviations from idealized norms (or forms): not only may a person be taken as diseased, but a tree, a society, a community, or a family. From this point of view, to call a phenomenon a disease is *always* to invoke cultural norms and to assert deviation from those norms.

Now, it seems clear that such deviations from cultural norms would from a God's-eye view, a detached spectatorial-contemplative view, or a view from nowhere, be merely one set of phenomena among the billions and billions of events constituting Nature, and would not be invidiously segregated from other phenomena of Nature as a qualitatively distinct category, requiring a special explanation. They become or are called *diseases* (and, yes, *defects, deficiencies, disruptions* or *disorganizations*—one can add a fifth *D*, *disorders*), not in terms of Spinoza's *sub specie eternitatas* or Kant's *Critique of Pure Reason*, but with respect to *human* social groups and the norms they have set up as desiderata to regulate human actions and transactions.

In such sociocultural contexts, in which purposes and interests are taken to operate in ways alien to the physical world, one is less concerned with determining the etiologies (causes) of such deviations from norms, or providing any systematic "theoretical" explanation which could "account for them" in the same set of terms that one uses for everything or anything else, than in *doing* something or *having something done* about them which will remove, remedy or cure them, restoring whatever it is that is taken to manifest them to normality (or "health").

One may claim to show, from a purely *theoretical* standpoint, that cancer is not a distinct phenomenon, qualitatively segregated in "nature" from other, "normal," bodily processes, and hence, from a physical point of view, not a disorder, disease, or other Big *D*; but when the practical concern is with restoring the entity or organism to some norm, such deviations are not conceived as merely natural variants, homogeneous in kind with others, but as *diseases*. *Disease* and its kindred, thus, may be taken to pertain not to the sphere of detached theory, where "all cats are grey in the dark," but to the sphere of interest-instigated and norm-regulated practice.

What is the upshot of all this? In any group presuming an ontology of things and processes, existing or subsisting independent of human acting and knowing, independent of human interest, any particular thing, entity or event that is putatively endowed with a *nature* or *essence*, could be taken as diseased (dis-ordered, dis-organized), relative to pure norms and forms taken as prior to individuals (Plato) or to potentialities inherent in individuals, which they would normally realize or actualize unless derailed by contingent factors or forces (Aristotle).

In such a society, the rage for order may be so pervasive that even the *deviations* from dominant, highly valorized norms for things, states, or events may themselves be hypostatized, and construed as having either one essence (nature), or assigned multiple essences (natures). Thus, we have such questions as: "What is the essence (nature) of illness? of psychosis? of depression? of schizophrenia? of dirt? of trash?" To be sure, these questions are often posed as "What is (the definition of) X?"; but insofar as "definitions" are tacitly or explicitly taken as a search for the discovery of *essences*, inherent in the "objects" or "entities," rather than "teleological weapons" (William James) to alter the map of our world, the presupposition is the same.

With the presumption of such a given ontology (or the way things are), one is also likely to take special groups, presuming, or taken, to be cosmically endowed, privileged, and legitimated to ferret out the signs of disease or to intervene in specified (often esoteric) ways to remove the "deviants," possessing or inhabited by the disease, or to "recycle" them so that they can once more secure a place in the harmonious cosmos they disrupted.

Once, however, there is the Decline and Fall of a *particular* House of Essence; once a cosmically engendered and sanctioned ontology, comprised of fixed forms—hierarchically arranged—is denied; once God is dead, all who seek to usurp the place and power of God as final authorities, or as ultimate arbiters of the way things are, are themselves subject to critique and questioning, then we can expect, either with dismay or glee, the kind of mythomachia/logomachia that is all around us today; indeed, and in which, in the schizophrenia conference the contributors to this book participated in an attenuated and properly civil way.

Of course, we all know that such struggles over the definition of the world can easily go beyond academic proposals for new world hypotheses or definitional refinements. How bitter and bloody such conflicts may become is obvious in even a cursory glance at the international scene; at the internecine wars inside a state; in instances where those who take themselves to be oppressed or marginalized by existing institutions have gained voice and power and have risen up against the prevailing order, its forms of rationalization, and its managers, experts and professionals.

It is, perhaps, to be expected that those dismayed by the Fall of a *particular* House of Essence—disoriented, confused or threatened with displacement or dispossession by the breakdowns of *Law* and *Order* (in all their manifestations)—will not "go gently into the night." Decrying the proliferation of Towers of Babel, they will attempt, in one form or another, to restore the God(s) who ordained and founded the now lost House of Essence.

Less anticipated, perhaps, but obvious via a modicum of historical reflection, is the fact that those "revolutionaries" who undermine a particular House of Essence are rarely advocates of *permanent revolution* or *unceasing critique*. Once they are in power, attaining hegemony under the banner of Freedom, Reason, Science or whatnot, they subtly institute a new House of Essence, even while decrying essences, and often insist that a new sovereign or class of rulers (scientists, experts, competent, credentialled professionals) be given the sole power and right to define what there *really* is; to regulate who may licitly have opinions and speak about important matters; to determine what constitutes *knowledge* and what opinion, etc., so as to preclude deleterious ambiguity, polyvocality, and polluted or pernicious disseminations. Thus Plato; thus Hobbes; thus our current foundationalists and absolutists.

There may even be some minions of this New Order, this new House of Essence, who will be particularly alert to what they take to be residues from the Old Order ("tradition"), to old orthodoxies which are now heterodoxies and even heresies; to concepts and doctrines they had hoped had been once and for all eradicated. It may even be expected that some of them, holier than thou, will complain that the New Order has not sufficiently purified itself; that it is still infected with too much of the *terministic screens* characterizing the Old. Let us get rid of any discourse allowing one to speak of Agents or Persons; of Purposes; of Causes, Motives or Reasons; of Actions initiated by Agents that are more, or other, than Movements; of Powers, Dispositions, or Capacities; of Diseases, Disorders, Defects, Deficiencies.

Such a *remapping of the ontological domain*, under the aegis of natural science inquiry, is likely to be of more than local significance; it will be seen—gleefully by some, catastrophically by others—as having repercussions and reverberations throughout our ontology. For a small coterie of emancipated souls (proponents of eliminative materialism, advocates for the demise of folk-psychology, some sociobiologists) it will be taken as a prognosis or prophecy of the *final solution*, the end of human beings and human culture as distinctive categories. Did not Horkheimer and Adorno remark on this ineluctable outcome in their *Dialectic of the Enlightenment*? Did not

Merleau-Ponty acutely observe that Science has no place for the category of *person*?

Some, not only less sanguine, but positively melancholic at this creeping metastasis of the ideology of natural science ("physicalistic reductionism," "scientism," "mechanism," "positivism," "Cartesianism") will, with Donne, Wordsworth, Yeats, bemoan the hegemony of the "new philosophy" which 'calls all in doubt,' which 'murders to dissect,' that unlooosens the center leading to "mere anarchy." Still others, emitting clarion calls for a *new contextualism*, a *new historicism*, a *new relativism*, a *new pluralism*, will seek to restrict or subordinate the scope and role of science as it is now generally understood. A few hardy souls might even suggest that, instead of taking *science* as a privileged, distinctive or divinely segregated activity, itself impervious to "scientific scrutiny," it be subjected, as all other human and cultural institutions are, to historical, cultural, economic, and political examination. Hoist on its own petard, so to speak.

I could go on to discuss and seek to dismiss the variety of new claimants to occupancy of the House of Essence, those who have asserted that they had discovered the foundations on which we could resurrect a stable world order, and provide a clear picture of the way things really are. But there is not the time/place for such an excursus. Nor is this the time/place to elaborate on the variety of arguments that have been raised about the inscrutability or opaqueness of reference; the gaps between the signs we inescapably use and any referent assumed to be directly designated by such signs; or the gap between the signifier and signified of any sign.

Without filling in these necessary linkages, I shall leap to the conclusion of this essay. It is, in my view, useless and hopeless—as well as a waste or time—to discuss whether there is something or nothing out there to which the terms *psychosis, schizophrenia, schizophrenic, reality, self, and identity*, correspond, to which they are adequate. Such a discussion is likely to lead to Piagetian collective monologues, or to those exciting exchanges in which one says, "Yes, it is" and the other says, "No, it's not."

In her fascinating work, *Unruly Practices*, Fraser (1989) suggests that we put a moratorium on talking about the *needs* of various groups and individuals, and begin examining, historically and currently, the *politics of need representation* and the correlative issue of the *politics of need interpretation*. (See here, among others, Aronowitz, 1988; Bayer, 1987; Brenkman, 1987; Cottom, 1989; Coulter, 1989; D'Amico, 1989; Dillon, 1988; Lincoln, 1988; Longino, 1990; Mailloux, 1990; Mitchell, 1990; Needham, 1983; Riley, 1988.)

It seems to me that we may all profit by extending Fraser's proposal to all of *our* terms and forms of discourse, focussing on the politics of representation and interpretation for all of our taken for granted terms, for all of the extensions of such terms, for all the semantic changes they suffer in different contexts and through the practices of different interested agents.

In such an examination, it is, of course *essential* (how could I avoid that word) that we look critically not only at the multifarious discursive practices of others, but also at ourselves (the presumed men and women of knowledge), and, particularly scrutinize how and why we, conflictively, and often rancorously, engage in trying to persuade others that the ways in which we propose *defining* the world are the ways which should be adopted by others.

It will surely come as no surprise that in my beginning was my end. I started out suggesting Burke as a guide—not the final authority—and I conclude by restating his questions in the form well known to newspaper reporters: with regard to any proposals that situations be defined in a particular fashion, one should, at the very least, ask: what, who, where/when, how and why. And, if one questions these "categories" or this *grammar of motives*, reapply them to those who propose them.

Additional source materials not directly cited in the text are included in the References below.

References

Achinstein, P. (1968). *Concepts of science.* Baltimore, MD: John Hopkins Press.

Arac, J. (1988). *After Foucault.* New Brunswick, NJ: Rutgers University Press.

Arieti, S. (1955). *Interpretation of schizophrenia.* NY: Brunner.

Arieti, S. (1959). "Schizophrenia: Other aspects; Psychotherapy". In S. Arieti, (ed.), *American handbook of psychiatry, 1.* NY: Basic Books.

Aronowitz, S. (1988). *Science as power: Discourse and ideology in modern society.* Minneapolis: University of Minnesota Press.

Baker, L.R. (1987). *Saving belief: A critique of physicalism.* Princeton, NJ: Princeton University Press.

Ballard, J.G. (1985). Manhole 69. In *Best short stories of J.G. Ballard.* NY: Washington Square Press. [First published, 1957].

Bayer, R. (1987). *Homosexuality and American psychiatry: The politics of diagnosis.* NY: Basic Books.

Bellak, L. (1979). *Disorders of the schizophrenic syndrome.* NY: Basic Books.

Berger, P. & Luckmann, T. (1967). *The social construction of reality: A treatise in the sociology of knowledge.* NY: Anchor Books.

Bergner, J. (1988) *The origin of formalism in social science.* Chicago: University of Chicago.

Bernstein, R. (1988). The rage against reason. In E. McMullin (ed.), *Construction and constraint*. South Bend, IN: University of Notre Dame Press.

Bleuler, E. (1969). *Dementia praecox or the group of schizophrenias*. NY: International Universities Press.

Bowers, M. (1974). *Retreat from sanity*. Hammondsworth: Penguin Books.

Brenkman, J. (1987). *Culture and domination*. Ithaca, NY: Cornell University Press.

Burke, K. (1935). *Permanence and change: An anatomy of purpose*. Berkeley: University of California Press.

Burke, K. (1945/1969). *A grammar of motives*. Berkeley, CA: University of California Press.

Burke, K. (1952). *A rhetoric of motives*. NY: Prentice-Hall.

Burke K. (1966). Language as symbolic action. Berkeley: University of California Press.

Burridge, K. (1979). *Someone no one: An essay on individuality*. Princeton, NJ: Princeton University Press.

Carrithers, M., Collins, S., & Lukes, S. (1985). *The category of the person*. New York: Cambridge University Press.

Cassirer, E. (1944). *The problem of knowledge. Volume 4*. New Haven, CT: Yale University Press.

Cassirer, E. (1953). *Substance and function and Einstein's theory of relativity*. NY: Dover Publications.

Cohen, F. (1954). The reconstruction of hidden value judgments: Word choices as value indicators. In L. Bryson, et al. (eds.), *Symbols and values: An initial study*. NY: Harper.

Cottom, D. (1989). *Text and culture: The politics of interpretation*. Minneapolis: University of Minnesota Press.

Coulter, J. (1989). *Mind in action*. New Jersey: Humanities Press International.

Crawshay-Williams, R. (1957). *Methods and criteria of reasoning: An inquiry into the structure of controversy*. London: Routledge & Kegan Paul.

Crews, F. (1963). *The Pooh perplex: A freshman casebook*. NY: Duttton Press.

Crookshank, F.G. (1923, 1946). The importance of a theory of signs and a critique of language in the study of medicine. Supplement II to Ogden, C.K. and Richards, I.A. *The meaning of meaning*. Harvest.

Crowcroft, A. (1967). *The psychotic: Understanding madness*. Harmondsworth: Penguin Books.

D'Amico, R. (1989). *Historicism and knowledge*. NY: Routledge Press.

David-Menard, M. (1989). *Hysteria from Freud to Lacan*. Ithaca, NY: Cornell University Press.

Dillon, G. (1988). *Rhetoric as social imagination*. Bloomington, IN: Indiana University Press.

Douglas, M. (1966). *Purity and danger*. London: Routledge Kegan Paul.

Douglas, M. (1982). *Natural symbols*. NY: Vintage.

Edelson, M. (1960). *The idea of a mental illness*. New Haven, CT: Yale University Press.

Feder, L. (1980). *Madness in literature*. Princeton, NJ: Princeton University.

Federn, P. (1952). *Ego psychology and the psychoses*. NY: Basics Books Press.

Felman, S. (1985). *Writing and madness*. NY: Cornell University Press.

Foucault, M. (1961). Historie de la Folie. Paris: Plon.

Fraser, N. (1989). *Unruly practices: Power, discourse, and gender in contemporary social theory*. Minneapolis: University of Minnesota Press.

Freeman, T., Cameron, J., & McGhie, A. (1958). *Chronic schizophrenia*. NY: International Universities Press.

Godzick, W. (1986). Introduction to De Man, P. *Resistance to theory*. Minneapolis: University of Minnesota Press.

Knapp, B. (1969). *Antonin Artaud: Man of vision*. NY: D. Lewis.

LaCapra, D. (1985). *History & criticism.* NY: Cornell University Press.

Lea, H.C. (1972). *The ordeal.* Philadelphia, PA: University of Pennsylvania Press.

Lea, H.C. (1973). *Torture.* Philadelphia: University of Pennsylvania.

Leitch, V. (1983). *Deconstructive criticism: An advanced introduction.* NY: Columbia University Press.

Lincoln, B. (1988). *Discourse and the construction of society.* NY: Oxford University Press.

Lloyd, G. (1989). *The man of reason: 'Male' and 'female' in Western philosophy.* Minnesota.

Loewe, M. & Blacker, C. (1987). *Divination and oracles.* London: Unwin.

Longino, N. (1990). *Science as social knowledge: Values and objectivity in scientific inquiry.* Princeton, NJ: Princeton University Press.

Lowe, M. & Hubbard, R. (1986). *Woman's nature: Rationalizations of inequality.* Pergamon/Athena.

Mailloux, S. (1990). Interpretation. In F.Lentricchia & T. McLaughlin (Eds.), *Critical terms for literary study.* Chicago: University of Chicago Press.

Margolis, J. (1990). The truth about relativism. In M. Krausz (Ed.), *Relativism: Interpretation and confrontation.* South Bend, IN: University of Notre Dame Press.

McCarthy, T. (1990). Scientific rationality and the 'strong program' in the sociology of knowledge. In E. McMullin (Ed.), *Construction and constraint.* South Bend, IN: University of Notre Dame Press.

McMullin, E. (1990). *Construction and constraint: The shaping of scientific rationality.* South Bend, IN: University of Notre Dame Press.

McNeill, J. (1956). *A history of the cure of souls.* NY: Harper Torchbooks.

Mendosa, E.L. (1989). *The politics of divination.* Berkeley, CA: University of California Press.

Michaux, H. (1974). *The major ordeals of the mind, and the countless minor ones.* NY: Harcourt Brace Jovanovich.

Mitchell, W.J.T. (1990). Representation. In F. Lentricchia & T. McLaughlin (Eds.), *Critical terms for literary study.* Chicago.

Needham, R. (1983). *Against the tranquility of axioms.* Berkeley, CA: University of California Press.

Northrop, F.S.C. (1944). *The logic of the sciences and humanities.* NY: MacMillan.

Ong, W.J. (1967). *The prescence of the world: Some prolegomena for cultural and religious history.* New Haven: Yale University Press.

Ong, W.J. *(1981).* Fighting for life: Contest, sexuality, and consciousness. Ithaca, NY: Cornell University Press.

Parkinson, G.H.R. (1968). *The theory of meaning.* London: Oxford University Press.

Pepper, S. (1970). *World hypotheses, a study in evidence.* Berkeley: University of California Press.

Perry, J.W. (1974). *The far side of madness.* Englewood Cliffs, NJ: Prentice Hall.

Rabinow, P. (1988). *The Foucault reader.* NY: Pantheon.

Rabinowitz, P. (1989). *Before reading: Narrative convention and the politics of interpretation.* Ithaca, NY: Cornell University Press.

Riley, D. (1988). *Am I that name?: Feminism and the category of 'women' in history.* University of Minnesota Press.

Robb, K. (1983). *Language and thoughts in early Greek philosophy.* Monist Library of Philosophy. La Salle, IL: Hegeler Institute.

Rosenbaum, B. & Sonne, H. (1987). *The language of psychoses.* NY: New York Universities Press.

Rosenfeld, H. (1959). *Psychotic states.* NY: International University Press.

Rorty, R. (1988). Is natural science a natural kind?". In E. McMullin (Ed.), *Construction and constraint.* South Bend, IN: Notre Dame University Press.

Ruitenbeck, H. (1975). *Going crazy.* NY: Bantam Books.

Sarbin, T. & Mancuso, J. (1980). *Schizophrenia: Medical diagnosis or moral verdict.* Pergamon.

Schilder, P. (1976). *On psychoses.* NY: International Universities Press.

Scull, A. (1981). *Madhouse, mad-doctors, and madmen: The social history of psychiatry in the Victorian era.* Philadelphia, PA: University of Pennsylvania Press.

Spurr, D. (1985). Colonialist journalism: Stanley to Didion. *Raritan, 5,* No. 2, 35-50.

Szasz, T. (1970). *Ideology and insanity: Essays on the psychiatric dehumanization of man.* Garden City, NY: Anchor Books.

Szasz, T. (1974). *Schizophrenia: The sacred symbol of psychiatry.* NY: Basic Books.

Turner, V. (1974). *Dramas, fields and metaphors: Symbolic action in human society.* Ithaca, NY: Cornell University Press.

Turner, V. (1967). *The forest of symbols.* Ithaca, NY: Cornell University Press.

Veith, I. (1965). *Hysteria: The history of a disease.* Chicago: University of Chicago Press.

Walker, D.P. (1981). *Unclean spirits.* Philadelphia, PA: University of Pennsylvania Press.

Weintraub, K.J. (1978). The value of the individual. Chicago, IL: University of Chicago Press.

16
Tunnel Vision and Schizophrenia
Robert C. Carson

Before proceeding with specific commentary on the immediately preceding chapters, I want to take the liberty of exploiting my position of "having the last word" to make some more general remarks on the current status of research on the schizophrenia construct. Much contemporary professional propaganda (e.g., Andreasen, 1984) would have us believe that a solution to the schizophrenia conundrum is just around the corner. My own view is that there is not the slightest chance of this happening at any time in the foreseeable future; that in fact our base of knowledge in scientific research on what we call schizophrenia is in almost hopeless disarray—owing in large part to a curiously perverse and apparently intensifying circumspection in the visions of most researchers in the field. Everything that we truly know about schizophrenia, in contrast, indicates the need for a comprehensive, contextualist view that allows for multitudes of interacting biological and psychosocial variables if we are ever going to achieve a satisfactory conceptualization of even the essential nature of the problem (Carson & Sanislow, in press).

Lest my title invite the speculation that I intend to propose yet another sign or symptom to aid in identifying those unfortunates deserving to be designated schizophrenic, I hasten to state explicitly that I find the phenomenon of tunnel vision far more reliably associated with the expert observers of the schizophrenia scene than with the human objects of their observations. Indeed, it has seemed to me that this particular "symptom" is at least as uniformly present among these observers, considered as a class, as is any symptom attributed to the class of persons we call schizophrenic. Without in any way impugning the motives, efforts or competence of the organizers of the conference on schizophrenia, I must say that my participation in this conference has afforded me an extraordinarily convincing but bittersweet confirmation of this heretofore only casually entertained hypothesis. My dominant impression of the conference, overall, was that of a group of highly intelligent and charmingly sociophilic persons largely unable to make intellectual contact with one another. The "epigenetic puzzle" (Gottesman & Shields, 1982) that is schizophrenia is unlikely to be solved so long as leading thinkers in the field, such as these conferees, can find no means of extricating themselves from an ideologically inspired paradigmatic dissonance that precludes the discernment of any overarching consensus.

As a group, the chapters by Professors Sarbin, Wiener, and Kaplan contain what may readily be seen as the most radical and controversial of the propositions advanced in this book. In its own way, each questions whether there *is* such a thing as schizophrenia, at least in the sense of there being empirical phenomena that closely match the purported entity normally denoted by the construct-term, that cannot be more parsimoniously addressed in other ways.

In my judgment, an appropriate level of skepticism of this sort serves the valuable function of reminding us that in more than a century of increasingly intensive research we have yet to unearth anything, at any level of observation (notably including the biological), that even approximates a core element or process invariantly associated with "schizophrenic" behavior. And despite all the reductionist hoopla about "astounding neuroscience advances," "the decade of the brain," and so forth, it is not, it seems to me, unreasonable at this stage to suggest that maybe it is just not there to be found. If so, a great many promissory notes of recent issue, emanating mainly from the biomedical community and involving huge sums of public money, will be defaulted on. It would have been better, I think, not to have made these promises in the first place. Having been made, however, they appear to have taken on a life of their own, one in which various incoherent, theoretically opaque, and quantitatively trivial (in terms of variance accounted for) findings are displayed with a fanfare more appropriate to major scientific advances, of which this enormously difficult field is, and most likely will remain, bereft. Appropriate scientific constraint and objectivity do not flourish in such a context, and it is refreshing when from time to time, as in these chapters, the Emperor's state of conceptual undress is uncompromisingly noted.

Professor Sarbin's chapter is not, as its title may suggest, merely another "schizophrenia as labeled social deviance" tract. Its real power, in my reading of it, resides in a sophisticated and well-researched attack on nothing less than the empirical foundations traditionally employed to support the construct of schizophrenia as a psychobiologic entity. To that extent, his argument has a crucially different focus from one limited to the often made, but still arguable, observation that craziness, like beauty, is entirely in the eye of the beholder (or the collective eye of a given culture). Sarbin engages his opponents, the neo-Kraepelinians, on their own turf with a litany of fatal and near-fatal flaws in the data base from which they operate. It is a virtuoso performance, albeit one certain to inspire outrage among True Believers of the schizophrenia doctrine—as indeed it did when its essentials were orally presented at the conference.

The chapter offered by Professor Wiener has the ring of a somewhat more traditional social science critique of the dominant psychiatric approach to the behavioral phenomena inspiring (within that approach) the schizophrenia rubric. In it he extends to the schizophrenia realm the same type of intriguing analysis he recently employed in discussing the phenomena of depression (Wiener, 1989). For both, he recommends that we try to understand these behavioral aberrancies within the same conceptual framework that we invoke for understanding more normative behaviors. In basic agreement with Sarbin, he suggests that these behavioral phenomena be viewed as purposive efforts at social transaction. Where these efforts appear "different," limited, imprecise, or otherwise ineffective, we should look to the individual's social history in relation to the present social context if we insist on identifying "causes" at all, rather than to presumed internally based "defects, deficiencies, disruptions, or disorganizations," i.e., to imputed "diseases."

I approach the obligation to fashion some remarks in response to Professor Kaplan's chapter with a degree of trepidation; one hardly knows how to take the statements of a conferee who declares the conference, at the outset, to be pointless, likening it to a "circus" or a "party," and even, by implication, to a gathering of conspirators. Its gadfly and revolutionary tone notwithstanding, however, the paper conveys a fundamental truth (dare I use the term?) none of us can afford to ignore. That truth has to do with the enormous power of duly constituted authority, in this case the mental health professions, to defame and nullify the social identity of those whose behavior upsets and perhaps implicitly holds up to ridicule an arbitrarily defined "natural order of things."

Needless to say in this context, Kaplan joins Sarbin and Wiener in finding the schizophrenia concept to be without empirical or rational substance; what he adds to their relatively apolitical analyses is an attribution of sinister intent, of illegitimate and systematic deployment of power to silence those who would challenge our collective sense of "reality." While none of the mental health professions can reasonably claim virgin status with respect to political Machiavellianism, my own impression is that Kaplan goes a bit too far here in reifying an interesting construction of facts that *could*, to be sure, signify massive conspiracy, but that need not. Actually, I think contemporary mental health professionals are as a group too confused, disorganized, and politically incompetent to be able to pull off anything even approaching the scenario that Kaplan, with appealing gusto and obvious relish, depicts.

As these three otherwise excellent works confirm, tunnel vision is not confined to those currently well funded biological types vainly searching for "schizophrenia" in molecular events occurring in the synaptic cleft, or in barely detectable (but statistically significant) brain deformities, of which at least some are doubtless the product of drug iatrogenesis. Tunnel vision occurs, as it does in this book, with distressing frequency in philosophical and social science critiques of the dominant psychiatric ideology of schizophrenia as brain disease.

Common to such critiques is a failure to give due recognition to the frequently devastating disruption of effective, self-affirmative living associated with the "diagnosis." These folks, by and large, are not merely eccentric, not merely romantic but inarticulate rebels rejecting the "system." Their deficits are very real and crippling; they *preclude* a mutually satisfactory engagement with the social environment, which for the most part is not so much rejected as it is perceived to be a hopelessly unfathomable morass with high potential for further psychic injury. The extraordinary naivete of the belief that some sort of medical magic bullet can be found that will reverse such a generalized dysfunction of the person as a social being does not, it seems to me, justify the conclusion that no disorder exists. From this perspective, I can appreciate the frustration psychiatrists experience when assailed with such arguments; according to the way our society is structured it is they, after all, who bear the brunt of the responsibility for "doing something" in the face of these profoundly disconcerting phenomena. One could wish, of course, that they display (again as a group) a level of humility more in keeping with the massively elusive problems they have taken on, but it must be more than a trifle maddening to hear repeatedly from the towers of academia that these problems do not exist.

Finally, I want to comment on the egregious imbalance that currently exists in funding for research on schizophrenia—another example of tunnel vision. I think down the road we shall pay a heavy price for our almost total neglect for more than a decade, of the psychosocial dimensions, both causal and restorative, of the disorders we call schizophrenic. No objective reading of the evidence we have in hand (see, e.g., Carson & Sanislow, in press) could possibly be taken as justifying this neglect. Perhaps, as Professor Kaplan intimated, there really is a conspiracy afoot; this one, however, I take to be more misguided by fantasies of imminent "great and desperate cures" (Valenstein, 1986) than sinister. It is a tragedy nonetheless, especially when we consider that we are training an entire generation of mental health professionals and researchers to be selectively blind to those psychosocial characteristics of their "schizophrenic" patients that remain as a bar to productive societal participation long after the "symptoms" of a given psychotic episode have abated or have been pharmacologically suppressed.

References

Andreasen, N.C. (1984). *The broken brain: The biological revolution in psychiatry*. New York: Harper & Roe.

Carson, R.C. & Sanislow, C.A., III (in press). The schizophrenias. In H.E. Adams & P.B. Sutker (Eds.), *Comprehensive handbook of psychopathology*, 2nd Ed. New York: Plenum.

Gottesman, I.I. & Shields, J. (1982). *Schizophrenia: The epigenetic puzzle*. Cambridge: Cambridge University Press.

Valenstein, E.S. (1986). *Great and desperate cures*. New York: Basic Books.

Wiener, M. (1989). Psychopathology reconsidered: Depressions interpreted as psychosocial transactions. *Clinical Psychology Review, 9*, 295-321.

17
Postscript: Premises and Positions
William F. Flack, Jr., Daniel R. Miller, and Morton Wiener

Looking back, we decided to devote this last chapter to premises, particularly those pertinent to philosophy of science. We did not originally anticipate that we would conclude with this topic, although it is prominent in three chapters and considered in most of them. To explain our reasons, we begin at the beginning.

We thought of holding this conference on schizophrenia because the topic is so important, and there is so much disagreement about it. True, most practitioners and some researchers adhere, more or less, to the standards defined in the Diagnostic and Statistical Manual (DSM) and other, similar systems. But anyone misled into thinking that there is a general consensus about the topic is readily disabused of that idea by a perusal of the literature and the papers in this volume.

Such disagreements have obvious consequences, particularly for the decisions made in the name of schizophrenia, which have a profound impact on the lives of millions of individuals diagnosed as schizophrenic throughout the world in terms of interventions, societal reactions, and legal consequences.

In the previous chapters, the conceptual issues are clearly drawn. One of the most important of these is the observation that there are so many toilers in what is considered, by and large, a common field of clinical activity and research, and yet precious few common terms and conceptions have evolved that would enable professionals to communicate with one another. Schizophrenia has been a subject of constant study to which a massive amount of time, effort, and fiscal resources have been dedicated. Almost one hundred years of effort, aimed at clarifying the figure and ground of the phenomena subsumed under this category, has resulted in far less clarity or immediate help than efforts in most other kinds of endeavor.

Many years have elapsed since there was a conference on the concept of schizophrenia as distinguished from the reporting of empirical findings. In addition, there has been a proliferation of publications that, in our opinion, have a bearing on the nature of the concept: empirical findings concerning genetic linkages, medical and philosophical analyses of the nature of disease, and sociological conceptions of madness are just a few of the topics researchers are investigating.

There are any number of publications on the nature of schizophrenia. Wouldn't this be a good time, we asked ourselves, to see if it was possible to survey the field and to assess its advances and problems? We did not want to prejudge the work of the conference. In fact, we each had our own biases, which we hoped to test in the crucible of common examination and criticism. In our invitation, therefore, we asked the deliberately vague question: What is schizophrenia?

We were not, of course, anticipating any clear-cut answers. We were hoping to learn about the basic problems that are of concern to specialists in the field. Many important issues were discussed during the conference. For instance, the issue of defining schizophrenia raises the more fundamental question of how one defines anything. That question immediately raises many subsidiary questions: Can there be one true definition? Is it implied that schizophrenia is something that exists, like the Eiffel Tower, or is it a concept that is used to conceptualize certain phenomena for particular purposes? We could go on and on with further clarifying questions, many of which the participants in the conference explored in creative ways. From differences in the answers to these questions, we hoped to derive some patterns in the thinking of a creative group of researchers with diverse backgrounds. In addition, we thought we might obtain some clues that would suggest why the creation of some kind of consensus has been such a refractory problem.

Weltanschauungen, Tunnel Vision, and Consensus

Just how successful the conference was in elucidating patterns of thought may be inferred from the preceding chapters. What interests us here is the manner in which the discussions developed. The papers were circulated beforehand. In the meetings, each paper was summarized by the author, and most of the time was then spent on the group's commentaries. From the beginning the styles of presentation tended to be confrontational. This was not surprising since we had invited people with a very wide range of viewpoints.

In a typical discussion during the conference, the group would make considerable headway in clarifying the implications of the paper being presented, but sooner or later the deliberations would end in gridlock. This was usually because doubts were being expressed about basic premises that the speaker regarded as self-evident. Often the participants divided themselves into groups whose opinions on various subjects tended to take predictable directions.

The problem arose early during considerations of the status of schizophrenia as a construct. One group of participants seemed convinced that schizophrenia is a pathological state, like any other disease, and that it originates in a biological predisposition. A second group accepted the designation of a pathological state, but emphasized that schizophrenia is only a term, with limited utility in depicting the nature of the state. Still others were willing to assume the existence of something like the problems subsumed under the concept of schizophrenia, but they took exception to some of its underlying assumptions. A final iconoclastic group doubted the value of the concept, and questioned whether there are empirical phenomena that corresponded to what the term implies.

Further spice was added to the proceedings by confrontations between conferees with seemingly irreconcilable differences. In his chapter, Kendell states, for example, that schizophrenia is a medical concept, questions the qualifications of non-medical professionals to evaluate it, assumes that most social scientists think of schizophrenia as simply a form of deviant behavior that can be explained away in terms of cultural background, limited vocabulary, and emotional arousal, and argues that genetic evidence is at the heart of the difference of opinion between psychiatrists and social scientists.

Taking up the challenge, Sarbin claims that systematic studies have failed to produce any determinate findings that justify the use of schizophrenia as a diagnostic entity, describes schizophrenia as a figment of the psychiatrist's disordered consciousness, and recommends that it be banished to the dustbin of history along with phlogiston, masturbatory insanity, and demon possession. Kaplan adds that schizophrenia is one of a set of discursive practices used by groups in power to "subjugate, subordinate, pathologize, medicalize, and, if possible or convenient, normalize ... those who deviate from the values and norms of a social order ..."

Such provocative statements were obviously not calculated to achieve the neutrality that is often prized in the ivory tower. In fact, the conference provided a disappointed Carson with a "bittersweet confirmation" of the hypothesis that tunnel vision is "far more reliably associated with the expert observers of schizophrenia than with the human objects of their observations." He cannot envision much progress so long as leading thinkers, such as members of the conference, are unable to extricate themselves from "an ideologically-inspired paradigmatic dissonance that precludes ... discernment of any overarching consensus ..."

Not everyone had this pessimistic impression. Some conferees were not sure that consensus is possible, or even desirable, at the present time, and felt it would be more appropriate to investigate the difficulties that diminish the possibility of consensus. During the conference, confrontation by participants with different ideologies often helped to clarify the reasons for the differences even when it did not lead to consensus. Moreover, it should be kept in mind that we were discussing systems of classification, a topic that usually engenders strong feelings. Kaplan describes such systems as "passionate proposals to construe the world in certain ways instead of others..." Like Margolis, Kaplan thinks that schisms among different groups go beyond philosophies of science; they involve divergences in "Weltanschauungen or orientations in which the very nature and status of what we take to be reality, knowledge, and science" are in dispute.

Styles of Thinking

The participants' differences in their interpretations of various kinds of evidence highlight the significance of particular styles of thinking. In Kendell's opinion, an assumption of biological differences is the core of the concept of schizophrenia. In his opinion, there is incontrovertible evidence that genetic factors play a major role in its etiology. In his account of etiology, Jaques makes no reference to genetic evidence. McHugh and Zubin think that the genetic evidence is suggestive. Claiming that there are no determinate criteria for identifying schizophrenia, Sarbin sees little purpose in studying the genetic etiology of a phenomenon he considers a social myth, and adds that the studies are riddled with methodological, statistical, and interpretational errors. Of primary relevance to this chapter is the problem posed by the fact that five eminent researchers disagree in their evaluations of some of the most carefully designed studies in the field.

A major problem noted by a number of participants (Miller & Flack, Kendell, Wiener) is raised by evidence that schizophrenia does not satisfy Bleuler's primary criterion that symptoms occur only and always in the clinically identified group. A number of disorders are included in the Diagnostic and Statistical Manual that, although they are classified as being different from schizophrenia, have some of its characteristics. Studies reveal the existence of schizophrenic symptoms in normal individuals and in patients with functional disorders that would not be expected to overlap with schizophrenia. Attempts to locate boundaries that would permit the discrimination of schizophrenia from other syndromes have been generally unsuccessful. Finally, patients diagnosed as schizophrenic do not have a common course of illness, nor do they respond similarly to the same treatment.

Coulter thinks that some criticisms are unwarranted. He advocates that a distinction be made between the use of the concept schizophrenia, in the clinical and in the research domains, and he thinks that the two uses were sometimes conflated in the discussions. He adds that there can be procedures for ruling out schizophrenia in certain cases, even though it cannot be identified with certainty. In addition, Coulter thinks that the existence of borderline cases does not, in itself, render all diagnoses useless. Nevertheless, he concludes that the continued use of the term is counter-heuristic, primarily because it cannot be demonstrated that subjects so diagnosed share a range of demonstrable, comparable properties. Carson, Sarbin, Wiener, and Kaplan agree.

As usual, the conferees are split, the most critical being members of non-medical disciplines. In a group that has a more sanguine outlook, all but one are psychiatrists. Most of them do not concern themselves with the value of schizophrenia as a concept; they just assume it. However, some reinterpret certain findings, and emphasize the complexity of the pathology. It is possible, for example, that there is a group of schizophrenias, each with its unique etiology, in which case some of the criticisms would be inappropriate (Kendell). When advocates of the concept do consider the empirical evidence, some admit that the data do not offer much support of the concept of schizophrenia as a disease. Nonetheless, they still insist that schizophrenia is a biomedical condition, and enthusiastically proclaim their faith in the use of disease as a heuristic model—the "single most successful method of approaching anomalies in physical disorders over the last centuries" (McHugh).

Levels of Analysis

We could have cited a number of other such schisms. As suggested by Margolis, Miller & Flack, Kaplan, and Wiener, they can be attributed, in part, to differences in premises that are usually viewed as part of the philosophy of science. Being premises they are neither right nor wrong. They are part of a weltanschauung that enables people to make the best sense they can about the world around them. Depending on one's preferences, however, such premises can have a profound effect on our definitions of concepts, our phrasing of questions, and our preferences for particular types of methods.

We begin with the predilection for a particular level of analysis. Kraepelin and Bleuler were guided in their thinking by a traditional medical model of disease. Each disease was regarded as a unique, natural phenomenon identified by its special pattern of signs and symptoms; its understanding required the identification of an agent, which was usually external. Disease was conceived as a configuration of signs, symptoms, and physiological laws pertinent to the nature of the agent. This position is described clearly in the chapters by Kendell and McHugh.

This conception of disease entails a commitment to *reductionism*. It assumes that what some take to be social and psychological phenomena are best explained by reanalysis into the concepts of biology, and further, if possible, into the concepts of chemistry and physics. This leads to a deemphasis of social and psychological findings in favor of physiological and biochemical ones. Complex social and psychological concepts are reduced into simpler, atomistic biological and chemical concepts that are presumably *universal* since they apply to structures and functions of the body that are independent of environmental, particularly cultural, conditions. McHugh, for example, follows the lead of Kraepelin and Bleuler in stating that schizophrenia is a disease. His reasoning depends in part on the assumption that its symptoms are manifestations of some structural or functional abnormality of a bodily part. He is confident that investigators of schizophrenia are likely to trace it to a specific brain disorder that is a necessary but not sufficient condition to produce the disease.

Most conferees are more comfortable working at the psychological level, though they usually venture into biological and cultural levels as well. Strömgren, for example, offers a psychopathological theory of schizophrenia whose core is autism. Autism, he thinks, is a defense mechanism that enables the person to survive intolerable idiosyncratic situations. Certain psychological events, he thinks, are necessary conditions for the development of schizophrenia; vulnerability to them may be increased by genetic predispositions or by brain pathology.

Some conferees who tend to think at the psychological level are firm in their opposition to reductionism. Strauss' intensive clinical studies reveal properties of psychological functioning that are inconsistent with the conception of a "broken brain." He doubts whether a simple cure for schizophrenia can exist; there are too many complex, interlevel, interactive processes at the very core of human mental functioning. In his criticism of reductionism, Margolis begins with the assumption that, as indicated in the DSM, schizophrenia involves disorders of cognition. Since cognition refers to the ways in which we organize our world conceptually, a theory of schizophrenia implies a philosophy of knowledge and a conception of the meaning of science. Cognition, he thinks, also implies a functioning self that is culturally and historically formed; disorders of this molar functioning cannot be reduced to somatic terms, and are not testable by the methods typically employed in the physical and biological sciences. Other arguments against reductionism are offered by Carson, Cromwell, Jaques, and Wiener.

Investigators who work primarily with somatic data expect their findings to apply in every society and historical period; a claim that Bleuler made about his concept of schizophrenia. Findings are not necessarily expected to be universal at the social level at which people interact in the family, at work, in the community, or as members of the larger society. Investigators who work with such data often postulate the emergence of qualities that are not present in psychological and somatic components, an assumption that rules out the possibility of reduction.

At the societal level, there is a considerable literature on psychosis in different societies. Fabrega contributes some helpful comments concerning central issues in this literature that bear on the analysis of schizophrenia. One is the distinction betwen form and content. Certain psychological functions (perception, affect, drive) are often regarded as universal, but their contents are usually culturally determined. He also proposes that distinctions be made between weak, strong, and radical forms of cultural relativism as they apply to the understanding of schizophrenia.

In the weak form, universalistic conceptions are accepted as veridical and appropriate. In fact, the investigator is often concerned with developing such pancultural generalizations. In the strong form, the tenets of scientific objectivism and physiological and biochemical propositions about schizophrenia are assumed, but allowance is made for the possibility that culture can have a powerful influence on the development of symptoms. In radical cultural relativism, cultures are regarded as being so different as to be incommensurable. It is assumed that somatic explanations of schizophrenia fall outside the domain of human symbolic behavior, and, as products of Western thought, have little relevance to non-Western cultures. Since it is presumed that the epistemologies of different societies cannot be compared, there can be no possibility of a universal science of persons, a goal that is itself a product of Western thought.

Kaplan goes even further when he states that the very objects of everyday actuality are anthropocentric, politico-culturally constructed, parochial entities that are part of a socially constituted ontology that may differ radically from other socially constructed ontologies. For example, for several participants, the concept of disease has meaning only with respect to human social groups and the norms they have set up as desiderata to regulate human actions and transaction. This way of thinking is consistent with radical relativism. Wiener, who has a somewhat different orientation, notes the highly acculturated biases that are likely to affect clinical interpretations, and observes that the kinds of psychosocial actions that have been identified as pathological have differed historically, and among socio-cultural groups in the same era.

Other Dimensions of World Views

The papers in this volume reveal predilections for still other ways of organizing one's conception of schizophrenia. One is a preference for either *static or dynamic* versions of phenomena. In classic accounts of the search for causes of disease, the investigator typically looks for a static sign that helps to account for the pathognomonic characteristics—particular structural or functional anomalies of body parts, genetic structures, or biochemical processes. The study of changing systems is not usually applied in such an analysis. A dynamic orientation, in contrast, leads to the analysis of systems consisting of many interacting functions that are constantly changing. Strauss, for example, postulates that schizophrenia represents a process of growing dysregulation, a destablizing system. It is a process that involves ebb and flow, function and dysfunction, occurring in the same person. Any variety of forces—social, psychological, biological—may cause a deviation which feeds into another, which can then amplify it, or even reverse it.

Given the complexity of such a system, both etiologies and sources of stability can occur at many points in the sequence of events. It is, therefore, not meaningful to look for the basic pathognomonic feature. Instead, one attempts to interpret a complex organization of changing features acting within the context of the person and interacting with biological and social systems.

Practitioners with dynamic orientations usually study the characteristics of their patients in great detail. M. Bleuler describes how his father sought to learn about the lives of his patients by working with them, playing and walking with them, even organizing dancing parties with them, and attempting to understand their whole inner lives. On studying his patients in comparable detail, M. Bleuler finds that schizophrenics have no characteristic dispositions, lose no particular functions for good, and reveal no characteristic course or outcome. He has come to think in terms of interacting systems in change, and to view schizophrenia as a disruption of "inner harmony." He thinks it highly unlikely that there is a specific cause.

Inherent in, but not necessarily associated with, dynamic analysis is a predilection for *temporal* analysis. The quest for pathognomonic signs is not usually aimed at clarifying processes that unfold over time; either there is or is not a lesion of the brain. This is less true when the subject of study is the socially functioning individual. From detailed studies of patients, Strauss infers that schizophrenia entails the existence of "...complex interactive processes with many component causes unfolding over time..." A sequential analysis of events may show that a problem leads to a minor deviation that feeds into another and is amplified by it, or possibly reversed by it; the changing sequence continues in the direction of either greater stabilization or destabilization. More specifically, the attention of a caring person or the availability of a job can set off a sequence beginning with the patient's increased activity that results in greater hope and self-esteem and diminished social isolation. These changes may intensify the relationship to the caring person, which, in turn, may facilitate the establishment of new social contacts. In this type of analysis, etiology consists of a complex pattern consisting of many changing components. The conception of a single pathognomonic feature precludes the analysis of constantly changing, interactive systems over time.

Cromwell employs temporal analysis to raise questions about the criteria for identifying schizophrenia. He begins with the observation that the developers of DSM-III decided to emphasize operational criteria obtained from the clinical interview, and to deemphasize their links to clinical decision making and prognosis. Reliability, for example, was assessed in terms of correlations between two or more clinical judges who viewed the same behavioral sample from one interview. The operational emphasis increased inter-judge reliability, Cromwell asserts, but not reliability based on consistency over time.

Cromwell thinks that the quest for operational criteria has led to a mistaken preference for Bleuler's accessory symptoms, and to the choice of positive instead of negative symptoms. Cromwell is critical because Bleuler's fundamental symptoms are basic and antecedent; they come first and are part of the essential configuration of the disorder itself. Accessory features follow, but not necessarily in every case. Choosing criteria primarily because they improve identifiability and reliability is unfortunate in that it does not avail itself of the important temporal analysis that might help in discriminating between the symptoms that are antecedent and consequent—a discrimination that can provide information relevant to validity.

Like Strauss, Cromwell believes that schizophrenia has a course long before, as well as after, the appearance of clinical pathology. Experiments suggest that some of the antecedent factors are deviations in attentional and information processing, which are salient among the offspring of schizophrenic parents, and may develop because of genetic-environmental factors affecting brain processes. Cromwell thus proposes a train of events that begins with genetic predispositions and early experiences. These contribute to a faulty processing of sensory and interpersonal information, which results in trauma and anxiety. These are succeeded by unidentified mechanisms which lead to manifest clinical features.

Another speculative sequence is used to explain the effectiveness of the combination of family therapy and pharmacotherapy. The train of events suggested by Cromwell begins with the patient developing negative symptoms, which the family condemns. The second step is initiated by prodromal symptoms, which the family also misinterprets. Next in line are the positive symptoms which elicit a mix of guilt, blame, denial, and criticism, thus elaborating the family's pathology and exacerbating the disorder. Family therapy, Cromwell asserts, helps to prevent relapse and neuroleptic therapy helps to diminish the positive symptoms.

There are still other predilections for ways in which knowledge can be organized, and which affected some of the positions taken in earlier chapters. Some researchers prefer to restrict their conceptions and questions to *phenotypes*, often overt behavior; others look for explanations in underlying *genotypes*, usually at a lower level. Some investigators will only consider *objective* evidence, while others concentrate on understanding the reports of *subjective* psychological experience. Some search for specific forms of pathology in their explorations of etiology; others reject this assumption of *discontinuity*, and, assuming a *continuity* in all behavior, investigate the vulnerabilities and traumatic events that can create pathological states in all of us. Some regard the schizophrenic individual as a *passive* object of a disease state that can befall virtually anyone; others view the symptoms as *active* attempts by the individual to make sense of a difficult environment and a traumatic history.

Specialists in the study of schizophrenia are not accustomed to identifying their preferences with respect to philosophy of science. In writing papers, most people seem to take it for granted that their viewpoints are shared by their colleagues. Preferences of the type described in this chapter tend to occur in clusters. Picture the confusion, even frustration, that occurs in a discussion between two individuals, one of whom thinks in molar concepts, is relativistic in interpretations of cross-cultural findings, and conducts minute-to-minute studies of patients' reports of their subjective states, on one hand; and another individual whose goal is a quest for a pathognomonic feature and who is most comfortable with reductionistic, objective, universally valid, and static concepts, on the other. There is no way of knowing, at this time, which orientations are most conducive to progress; it likely depends on the problem. We think that a giant step will have been taken when workers in the field of mental health become accustomed to examining the import of their philosophical premises for particular kinds of clinical theory and research.

Index